Praise for

# Own Your Self

"Kelly Brogan engages us in a courageous conversation about the epidemic of mental health issues in our society. Her work is an important part of the understanding that will set us free, at a time when an increasingly narrow interpretation of why such issues exist—and what we need to do to heal them—is as much a part of the problem as part of the solution."

— **Marianne Williamson**, *New York Times* best-selling author of *A Return to Love*

"We are in an age where mental, emotional, and physical balance has become our highest value. *Own Your Self* gives you the best possible solution on how to change your mind, your body, and your life. Kelly Brogan, M.D., does an amazing job combining cutting-edge information along with the practical tools for you to live a healthier personal reality. Her clinical and holistic approach from years of experience in doing independent research as a successful psychiatrist will teach as well as inspire you to get real, get well, and get free. This book holds the keys to inner peace and true happiness."

— **Dr. Joe Dispenza**, *New York Times* best-selling author of *You Are the Placebo: Making Your Mind Matter*

"*Own Your Self* is as compassionate as it is radical. Kelly Brogan calls you to make a change more profound than you ever thought possible—and gives you a supportive, insightful road map to guide you every step of the way."

— **Shefali Tsabary**, Ph.D., *New York Times* best-selling author of *The Conscious Parent* and clinical psychologist

"Dr. Kelly Brogan is a voice of sanity and compassion for our healing crises. She sings into the heart of our buried wisdom, makes clear what's broken in the culture. And backing it with science, Kelly gives us the path to genuine healing and sovereignty. This is so hopeful. I want every woman to read this—and heal."

— **Danielle LaPorte**, creator of *The Desire Map* series

"If you want to work on releasing suppressed emotions, Dr. Brogan has given you the perfect guide in *Own Your Self*. She encourages you to listen to and honor your emotions—and any related physical symptoms—fully and deeply, so that you may find a permanent, healing solution that gets to the root of the problem."

— **Kelly Turner, Ph.D.**, *New York Times* best-selling author of *Radical Remission*

"Kelly Brogan's quest for truth has uncovered yet another priceless gem. This book is a road map of relief for those yearning for authentic self-acceptance and long-lasting emotional freedom."

— **Matt Kahn**, author of *Everything Is Here to Help You*

"This book is sourced in a deep and coherent spiritual radicalism. If you or someone you love is grappling with so-called psychiatric disorders, it is a potent instrument of intellectual liberation and practical healing."

— **Charles Eisenstein**, author of *The More Beautiful World Our Hearts Know Is Possible*

"*Own Your Self* is an education and a medical reformation—a much-needed island of sanity in a crazy world! Kelly Brogan is a true psychiatrist, a doctor of the soul, and a guide back home to your authentic self. Her synthesis of science, deep humanity, and practical tools for well-being are crystal clear and right on target. She empowers us all to unleash the power of self-care to bring wholeness and healing."

— **Joan Borysenko, Ph.D.**, *New York Times* best-selling author of *Minding the Body, Mending the Mind*

"Kelly Brogan has, once again, boldly, dangerously, and clearly pushed the conversation forward on how we individually and collectively heal. *Own Your Self* is at once an ice bucket over the head and a warm hug calling us home to the truest versions of ourselves, and then leading us there. I am elated to have this work to refer to from here forward."

— **Kimberly Ann Johnson**, author of *The Fourth Trimester*

# Own Your Self

## Also by Kelly Brogan, M.D.

*A Mind of Your Own*

*A Time for Rain*

# Own
# Your
# Self

The Surprising Path beyond Depression,
Anxiety, and Fatigue to Reclaiming
Your Authenticity, Vitality, and Freedom

## KELLY BROGAN, M.D.
### with Nancy Marriott

**HAY HOUSE, INC.**
Carlsbad, California • New York City
London • Sydney • New Delhi

*Published in the United States by:* Hay House, Inc.: www.hayhouse.com®
*Published in Australia by:* Hay House Australia Pty. Ltd.: www.hayhouse.com.au
*Published in the United Kingdom by:* Hay House UK, Ltd.: www.hayhouse.co.uk
*Published in India by:* Hay House Publishers India: www.hayhouse.co.in

*Cover and interior design:* Nick C. Welch
*Indexer:* Joan Shapiro

**Cataloging-in-Publication Data is on file at
the Libarary of Congress**

Hardcover ISBN: 978-1-4019-5682-0
e-book ISBN: 978-1-4019-5683-7
e-audio ISBN: 978-1-4019-5684-4

10   9   8   7   6   5   4   3   2   1
1st edition, September 2019

Printed in the United States of America

SUSTAINABLE
FORESTRY
INITIATIVE
Certified Chain of Custody
Promoting Sustainable Forestry
www.sfiprogram.org
SFI-01268
SFI label applies to the text stock

*To my beloved, Sayer, and to our fierce love that created the container and continues to provide the alchemical ingredients for my rebirth in this lifetime, so I may serve the liberation of human consciousness and reclamation of unconditional love for myself, my daughters, and every person who hears the call to come home.*

# CONTENTS

# INTRODUCTION

## From a Doctor of the Soul

When I went into psychiatry, attended MIT and Cornell University, never did I imagine that I'd come to shun the primary tool of my trade—namely, pharmaceuticals.

But that's exactly what I did. In 2010 I laid down my prescription pad, and I have not started another patient on prescription medication since. Instead, I now take a holistic approach to helping people overcome their most crushing struggles, including those labeled as generalized anxiety, bipolar disorder, and major depressive disorder.

The term *psychiatrist* means "doctor of the soul," and in today's world, millions of individuals are seeking their own souls—to feel alive, real, and strong—*to feel like themselves*. But they most often land in the office of a doctor who is trained to provide a singular service: a pill prescription. In fact, part of my training in conventional Western medicine was to dismiss and discount anything that's not scientifically measurable, which of course includes the spirit—the soul of a human being.

If people manage to avoid prescription medications, it's likely that they instead self-medicate with whatever they can find to temporarily ease the burden: recreational drugs, alcohol, sex, food, online shopping. All the while, they feel worse than ever, trapped outside of their own authentic selves.

How did we get here?

We have been told a story about illness: that it is caused by bad luck and bad genes, and that the best we can hope for is to survive it, mainly by leaning on prescription medications that too often have adverse effects or are just plain ineffective. But as new science and real stories of radical health reclamation light up the Internet, we are all beginning to see that story as old, limiting, and false.

Today, we know that we can adapt and change in real time. It's the beauty of epigenetics and the microbiome—a dynamic ecosystem within our bodies that presides over our well-being. I know that I can help people reclaim their vitality within the space of a few months, despite a lifetime of living out of alignment. All I do in clinical practice is work to restore the signal of safety for my patients. I use this phrase often—"signal of safety"—in reference to the many ways we can tell our nervous system that *It's okay, all is well, you can rebalance now.* And it is possible to do, and quickly, because the body longs for it that much.

This book is about a new story, the chief points of which I will cover in depth throughout the upcoming chapters, including:

- That your "mental" problems, such as fatigue, brain fog, depression, anxiety, and even mania and psychosis, are telling you to change your life, pointing the way for how to recover and recalibrate. Illness is a part of healthfulness because your psychospiritual baggage is part of your breakthrough.

- Why most people today live in a state of chronic fear and have lost the part of themselves that accepts—embraces and copes naturally with—uncertainty, pain, sadness, grief, loss, despair, and disappointment. There is a general malaise in our culture. People feel "homesick": they are missing feeling at home in themselves, in their communities, and in the fabric of society as a whole.

I also provide a light in the darkness. In order to know what you want and where you're going, you need to understand, feel, and see your possible destinations. You need to know that radical healing is possible. Radical healing was possible for Cindy, who resolved her 18 years of lupus symptoms in weeks, and for Ali, who put bipolar disorder behind her in months. Throughout this book, I'll introduce you to the people who will light the path that you deserve to walk. You'll hear their stories and read their words, taken directly from their communications to me during or after participating in the special program you'll learn about in this book. You can also find their stories on video on my website, in the Video Testimonials section.

How did they do it? They did it *themselves*. We have collectively moved beyond the era of the doctor-master-guru and into a phase of medicine where each individual has the opportunity to reclaim their own power to heal themselves, ideally in a community of support. In my first book, *New York Times* best-selling *A Mind of Your Own*, I spoke to women about healing depression. Here, I broaden the scope, speaking to all, and not just about depression, but about the struggle with illness in general and the negative mindset that leaves you living half a life, dependent on meds of all varieties. It turns out that there is a belief system required to escape that cage, and I'd like to help you engender it.

You'll also learn the core of my self-led Vital Mind Reset (VMR) online program, a "prescription" for diet and lifestyle change that is working for thousands to not only resolve the root cause of so-called mood disorders but help people get off medications they felt were theirs "for life." You'll hear from participants in the program—called Resetters—who are just like you, and have walked this path to share their wins, insights, and aha moments. Once you're on board with the reality of the situation I present in Part I: Get Real, about how psychiatric illnesses, including depression, are a summons to explore what is out of balance, from the physical to the psychospiritual, you'll be ready for Part II: Get Well, where I introduce you to a one-month dietary "Reset" program based on my clinical approach with patients one on one. Then, in Part III: Get Free, I'll guide you with practical tips and advice to take an inventory of what does not work in your new life and how to align more powerfully with what does work in regard to your beliefs about yourself and your health; your relationships with family, romantic partner, community; your orientation to the medical system; and your choice of work or career. The final freedom is developing trust in the universe and cultivating a perspective that can unleash abundant reserves of positive energy, a true *quantum shift* in how you live.

## YOUR OWN JOURNEY

Your journey begins when you submit to the reality of your circumstances, look at them and say, *okay.* You accept and surrender, raise the white flag, and stop fighting. Healing is a process of reunion with your body, your soul, and your environment. Resistance, and specifically a victim mindset, will just perpetuate the experience of sickness.

Almost every single one of my patients, at some point, looks at me and says, "I don't even know who I am anymore." Everything has changed, and the healing journey is surrender to the process of change. Sometimes the things that go wrong in our lives, including physical illness, happen when we have refused change at the point when it is most called for: when we continue to commute to an unfulfilling job, ignore the pain of a toxic relationship, or perpetuate a self-harming habit; when we refuse to stop what we're doing even when we do not feel well doing it; when we neglect to ask ourselves, *What's the matter?* or to turn a sympathetic ear to the reply.

It is a critical distinction that the doctor says, "Your machine is broken"; the shaman says, "You have fallen out of relationship with the whole"; and the Helper says, "Your illness is an existential question that ultimately you must answer."

I no longer think of myself as a doctor. Instead, I have come to see my role as that of the Helper, one who is, in the words of Marc Ian Barasch, author of *The Healing Path*, who coined the term, "a facilitator of self-discovery; a change agent helping to pry the patient loose from pathological life patterns; a helper urging him away from mere normalcy toward authentic being."

Such a role is not for the faint of heart. It's also not for those who are in it to fix everything and pack things away into tidy diagnostic categories and discrete outcomes. While suicidal patients have told me that I saved their lives, I suspect that the way in which they meant it is figurative, acknowledging too minimally their own readiness to change.

In fact, with the humbling success of my online Vital Mind Reset healing program, I have become convinced that right now, it simply takes strategic support and a loving community to catalyze the emergence of an individual's latent gifts and self-expansion.

## THE BEST WAY OUT IS THROUGH

My most urgent message is about the commitment you must make in order to benefit from the lessons in this book. That commitment is this: put your self-care *first*, and do that every day. From that space, everything gets clear, and you find yourself the protagonist in the adventure of your most beautiful life.

The path gets ever simpler and easier when you commit to your self-care. You shed what needs to go because the pull toward your most authentic self becomes too great. You find out where you have been donating your much-needed energy—what old constructs of safety have been leaching parts of you that are required for full integration. It will become clear what has to be reconfigured once you surrender to the unfoldment and accept the possibility that you are simply here to dance with life, not manage it, script it, or commandeer it. We think we want to be wealthy, attractive, intelligent, talented—but really, don't you just want to be yourself, comfortable in your own skin?

In this book, we will explore the surprising path to living a med-free life through a deep appreciation of the meaning behind your symptoms. Our experiences reflect what we need to accept, acknowledge, and transform in order to truly become our adult selves. Only when we embrace our experiences can we begin to live a healthful, natural life without relying on substances and a mindset that rob us of our true power. All it takes is a commitment to curiosity, and it is my sincere hope that this book will inspire this life-changing shift.

It's time to get real, get well, and get free! Let's begin.

# PART I

# GET
# REAL

Chapter 1

# CANARIES IN THE COAL MINE

*It is no measure of health to be well adjusted*
*to a profoundly sick society.*

— Jiddu Krishnamurti

When was the last time you felt deep despair? The last time you dealt with debilitating grief, uncontrollable sorrow, or paralyzing anxiety? You might have felt stuck, detached, confused, foggy—basically dead inside. You may have started to think there was something seriously wrong with you, something that might require medical attention.

Maybe you saw a doctor who lovingly handed you a prescription to "take the edge off," you watched a convincing commercial that promised relief, or you heard a friend tell you that she was "worried" about you and how you were doing.

Look around you. You are not alone. Pain and hopelessness pervade our world. If the description you just read doesn't fit you, it probably fits someone you love or are close to. People have a growing sense that something *just isn't right*. If you were to ask a room full of men and women if they think we are in the midst of an intensely disturbing time in human history, you'd see a lot of hands go up. And if you were to ask that same group if they've considered or tried (or are taking) medication for their pain, you'd also see a lot of hands raised.

I've come to see those people as the proverbial canaries in the coal mine sending a signal to everyone else about something that is very, very wrong. Exactly what it is that is so wrong, and why some people are more aware of it than others, I'll explain shortly, but first, let's take a look at the territory.

We are suffering, and the solutions we are presented with seem to be falling short. According to the 2016 National Survey on Drug Use and Health, 18.3 percent of adults live with a mental illness (44.7 million). That's nearly one in five. Women have a higher prevalence than men, and 18- to 25-year-olds have higher prevalence than older adults. Mood disorders, including major depression and bipolar disorder, are the third most common cause of hospitalization, costing $193.2 billion in lost earnings per year.[1]

While such stats seem to identify the problem, they also point to the source of the problem: modern medicine's rush to judgment in legitimizing conditions that may actually be driven by the very viewpoint that is reflected in these reports. Investigative journalist Robert Whitaker helped us recognize, in his groundbreaking book *Anatomy of an Epidemic,* that we are in the midst of a disability epidemic that is perpetuated by the very medications prescribed to treat anxiety, inattention, psychosis, depression, and mood instability.

Why are so many of our illnesses chronic and often resistant to the medications prescribed to help them? Is there something else going on that we are not aware of, and could it be that the symptoms so many of us experience are really a message, a warning even, that we must shift our perspective and embrace a bigger—and truer—picture than what conventional medicine has been showing us?

A new perspective involves a more complex and sophisticated view of the human body, mind, and soul. This view challenges our very concept of disease and illness, offering an understanding that is more empowering than what we've had before. We are learning that beliefs, cultural conditioning, and our interaction with our environment are the true determinants of health and illness. And, in fact, that genes are merely a suggested template.

In this chapter I'll be introducing you to that new view and set the course for the rest of the book to explore a radical way for you to respond to your experience of mental and physical suffering—and find that the two are inextricably linked.

## THE PROBLEM OF YOU

In order to understand a radically different perspective on the struggle so many are experiencing (and the transformation of struggle that this book presents), we need first to look at how conventional medicine has viewed illness. Sadly, through the lens of modern medicine, symptoms associated with "mental illness" are seen as a problem with *you*, and specifically with your brain chemistry. It is your genes that caused a brain chemical imbalance, you've been told: a problem of faulty wiring in need of management. You are the problem, and drugs are the answer.

But let's look closer. What follows from this view that the problem is with you and your brain chemistry is the belief that those who suffer from "mental illness" are the *victims* of their pathology. After all, you can't be responsible if factors outside your control are causing the symptoms. The medical profession and pharmaceutical companies rally around these helpless "victims" with campaigns to destigmatize mental illness, delivering the message: *It's not your fault. It's your brain chemistry, and there's nothing you can do about it.* But in this way, we keep millions captive to a narrative that disempowers and depersonalizes their very real experience.

I'm going to suggest a different perspective, one that is more in sync with a newly emerging view of the body and mind that you'll be learning about later in this chapter and throughout this book. For starters, the problem is not you, and those who are seen as victims are not victims but messengers of something important we need to pay attention to.

From my observations in over a decade of private practice, I've come to believe that those labeled as mentally ill are, in fact, the canaries in the coal mine, sounding an alarm with exquisite sensitivity in service of the rest of us. Their symptoms, including fatigue, insomnia, ceaseless unrest and worry, disconnection, and deep sadness, carry the message of unrecognized physical, emotional, and even spiritual factors. They are telling us all that something is missing, very "off," and we need to wake up and pay attention to find it and correct it in order to survive and be happy.

As the canaries in the coal mine, their bodily mechanisms are sensitive to toxicant exposure, processed foods, and otherwise industrial lifestyles, as much as they are sensitive to many other layers of wrongness unfolding on our planet today. Seen as part of a bigger picture, their "illness" is really a statement, a whole body/mind/soul refusal to accept what is wrong as normative.

Psychiatry as it is practiced does not acknowledge that something is really wrong, missing, or meaningfully imbalanced on this planet or in your life, beyond unfounded theories of brain chemistry (I will explore in Chapter 3 just how unfounded these theories are!). In fact, in the current system, the context of your experience is largely irrelevant to the psychotropic-prescribing clinician because your symptoms are a problem to be fixed, not a meaningful response to explore. The prevailing view is that symptoms like withdrawal, fatigue, apathy, and anxiety emerge from faulty wiring that requires a soldering patch.

But these symptoms aren't a problem with you; rather, they are signs of a sensitivity you possess. A sensitivity to *very real* factors and variables—from physical to spiritual. Something else is going on, and medicating the evidence of this sensitivity is like attempting to turn off the smoke alarm while letting the real fire rage.

## EVOLUTIONARY MISMATCH

Yes, something is profoundly off in our lives on this planet today. In fact, many things are acutely amiss: we are living disconnected from our bodies through an education system that primes us for industry; disconnected from our communities thanks to technology and isolated, single-family homes; and disconnected from the environment because of several centuries of science that says nature is a collection of utilitarian resources that will ultimately be successfully dominated by mankind. Furthermore, we are disconnected from our very souls by a dominant belief system that says you are only what you can produce, and disconnected from the mysterious wonder of the human experience by the worship of scientific dogma that says something only exists if we can measure and quantify it.

We come into this world through women who are told to be afraid of their birthing bodies while they drink Coke and eat McDonald's and fathers whose sperm marinated in trans-generationally disruptive pesticides. We are ultrasounded in the womb regularly, birthed surgically, formula-fed, vaccinated, left by mothers who have a three-week maternity leave, schooled into a state of near-irreversible brainwashing while being microwaved by 5G networks. As adults, we work jobs that mean nothing and take everything and engage in relationships that could never possibly heal all of the unexamined wounds we bring to them, all the while swimming in a bath of chemicals.

The true scope of our wandering from the path of right living is obscured by multi-billion-dollar industries that are invested in meeting our primary needs with superficial satisfactions. Such satisfactions never do meet our true needs but rather increase the symptoms of what is being labeled "mental illness."

*It is difficult to get a man to understand something when his salary depends upon his not understanding it.*

— Upton Sinclair

We have strayed so far from the path that there is a scientific phrase to capture our situation: *evolutionary mismatch*. This concept holds that we have evolved to have certain needs—physical, sensual, nutritional, relational—that are nonnegotiable according to our basic design. We are living a lifestyle—diet, stress level, movement and sunlight deficiency, toxic exposures, pharmaceuticals—that is incompatible with what our genome has evolved, over millions of years, to expect. When these very basic needs are not met, the body, mind, and spirit rebel.

One example is how we treat babies in our culture, ignoring how they are designed, expectant of and singularly oriented toward human skin-to-skin contact. In indigenous living, and throughout ancestral time, babies are held from the moment they are born until they can crawl (six to eight months) and are not left without human contact for one minute. It certainly is not a life begun in a sterile, quiet bed, alone in a nursery. Immediate skin-to-skin contact is so embedded in the evolutionary mother-newborn dyad that in the absence of this imprinting (in a hospital birth where the baby is whisked off for cleaning and testing), a mother's physiology begins to prepare for the grief of a stillborn, potentially contributing to anything from poor milk supply to a diagnosis of postpartum depression.

The latest effort to manage the increasing preponderance of women struggling after childbirth is a drug called brexanolone. After only three randomized trials including a mere 247 women, the drug has an unknown mechanism of action, unknown effects on breastfed infants, and a $20,000-to-$50,000 treatment price tag. Because of the drug's risk profile, a woman must receive the 60-hour intravenous infusion under medical supervision and cannot function as her infant's primary caregiver during that time. We can certainly do better by these women who are simply expressing a very real mismatch of their needs with what our society reflexively offers.

Evolutionary mismatch includes sociocultural factors as well as the myriad ways in which we expect our bodies to conform to the industrial era, such as:

- Genetic modification of foods
- Pesticides
- Processing of foods into food-like products
- Industrial chemicals
- Radioisotopes from nuclear energy
- In-hospital births
- Formula feeding
- Fluoridated water
- Electromagnetic pollution

- Vaccination
- Antibiotic and other pharmaceutical exposures
- Indoor living
- Sedentary lifestyle
- Isolated nuclear family living

So we must ask: Is depression (or any chronic illness) and our painful struggle with modern life an illness—or is it a logical response to a world that is "off" and to our experience that doesn't align with our role in the natural world—an evolutionary mismatch?

Today, as I said in the introduction, we know that we can change in real time—and we can do it quickly, because the body longs for alignment.

As long as we live against the body, however, the struggle will continue.

## THE CAGED ARTIST WITHIN

I think of those who feel this mismatch most keenly, those who are warning us by their very symptoms of what is off, as the *artists* among us. I use the term "artist" not in the traditional way but to refer to the sensitive creatives who feel their mismatch to the world and to their bodies as a sign that they don't fit.

Today, creative expression takes a backseat in our consumer-driven, productivity-oriented culture. Just as religion has become a dogmatic version of what it once was—a celebration of the experience of ecstatic merger—art has been neutered of its true power. That power lies in shedding blinders, lies, tales, and false identities and exposing the raw beauty in simply witnessing existence.

When artists are in alignment, they can channel direct experiences that shatter the frameworks that bind us into submission. They can come back to tell us about what they experienced, and in the sharing, the possibility increases that we too might have these experiences of wonder. It is only when they are forced to conform to today's societal expectations that they are pathologized, marginalized, and generally diminished. They may very well not even sense that something is missing, but the pain and suffering they experience *is* that sign. They live under a constant barrage of inadequacy, seeming failure, and "otherness" as they strive to force their square selves into the circular holes of Western culture.

Illness is often a reminder that the real you needs to be born from the ashes of your struggle. It is an invitation to address the false self that you are representing as the real you. The real you is the artist, the creative aspect of yourself, and it is not free.

Maybe your depression, chronic fatigue, attention deficit hyperactivity disorder (ADHD), and chemical sensitivity are just ways your body, mind, and soul are saying *no*. The demands of this world, the day-to-day experience of this food, these chemicals, this disconnection—it is all not working. Consider that your *no—your symptom*—is a reminder to yourself that there is another way. It's an invitation back to who you really are and to freeing your caged artist to become a greater expression of yourself.

## PRICKLES AND GOOS

The patients I work with, the people most likely to find themselves labeled with "mental illness" of one sort or another and recover through my program, are these artists, these sensitive souls responding to a sick planet. But what is it about them that is different from others?

Under the guidance of my mentor, the late Dr. Nicholas Gonzalez, I came to understand the bigger picture of how and why people get sick and recover in different ways. He showed me how the success of my particular dietary template (which you will learn about in Chapter 6) is the result of my primarily treating patients who are what he called *parasympathetic dominants*.

To understand that term, you'll need to know that the parasympathetic nervous system is an arm of the autonomic (think *automatic*) system that manages rebuilding, healing, and regenerating. It's sometimes referred to as the "rest and digest" system. Immunity, digestion, and elimination are managed by parasympathetic nerve function. When the parasympathetic nervous system is unbalanced, in states of dis-ease and stress, it becomes overactive, causing symptoms of apathy, fatigue, autoimmunity, allergy, weight gain, low thyroid and sex hormone function, and liquid cancers. You feel "tired but wired," and are likely to reach for your meds, your substances, and extra cups of coffee, even though they make everything worse.

Dr. Gonzalez explained to me that such parasympathetic dominants have typical traits that are amplified when they are under stress and eat the wrong diet. They are not hungry in the morning and "hangry" if they go too long without eating. They look at a piece of toast and gain weight. They are night people and don't get going until noon. They sweat, have loose stools, and suffer from allergies. Their skin flushes easily, and they crave fatty foods. They often have low libidos and low drive in general, and are often called "dreamers." These are the folks, Nick said, who are the "right brainers"—the Hemingways, Faulkners, and Picassos.

Broad sketches of these types may be familiar: there are alphas and betas, Type As and Type Bs, gunners and creatives, and my favorite, what philosopher Alan Watts called *prickles* and *goos*. Goos are the natural artists, the parasympathetic dominants, and the canaries in this coal mine of modern life who are telling us that things just ain't right.

This book is for you, the goos.

It's you, the goos, the parasympathetic dominants, who are being diagnosed with ADHD, chronic fatigue, depression, and multiple chemical sensitivity, and your time has come to awaken to your gift through reclaiming your health. You are responding correctly on a mind, body, and soul level to the wrongness of your lived experience. Your depression is a sign of this mismatch: it's a sign that the processed food and the 100,000 unstudied chemicals are not right for you. Your body is saying no. Your spirit is rejecting a lifestyle that prizes productivity, linear thinking, measurable achievement, and relentless application of will to subdue any obstacle. Your very soul is saying no to a life lived by punching the clock until you die.

Where does your life force go when you suffer from this mismatch? Too often, it goes into self-medication with alcohol that temporarily dampens the pain of disconnection, and often into prescribed medications that hijack consciousness.

Graham Hancock speaks about such legal instruments of mind control and the suppression of the kind of creative drive that would overturn our social structure. Perhaps, he says, this is why hallucinogens, despite their completely nonaddictive profiles, are banned.[2] The primal connection to metaconsciousness brought about by plant medicines such as *ayahuasca* could be the most threatening of all human behaviors to society as we know it.[3]

## HEALING THE ARTISTS

Ethnobotanist, mystic, and author Terence McKenna stated, "Artists are here to save mankind."[4] And it has become clear to me that healing the parasympathetic dominants, the goos, the canaries in the coal mine will save us all. As I facilitate the reclamation and recovery of one patient after another from psychiatric medication injury, from environmental and dietary poisoning, and from a fear-based attachment to a lifestyle that doesn't fit them, they show me that in this free state of self-possession, anything is possible. Their creativity blooms. They free that inner artist.

It's been my experience that physical healing is a portal to such transformation. My patients wake up to themselves when they are able to reclaim their agency through simple interventions like a clean diet. They blow the dust off their existence, and their inner compass comes back online. They expand and expand and expand in fearlessness, and bloom into visionaries.

If I can give you, the goos, the tools to balance your bodily organism, I believe you will come into fuller contact with your soul, your reason for being, and your essential role in ushering the rest of humanity into the next story.

You will find out what you are here to do. You will keep looking for it until you cannot control the drive to pursue what feels like the most important thing on the planet for you. This unstoppability is the hallmark of the creative life force.

As such a creative force, your freed artist within is the ambassador to the next story. It is you who will demonstrate what it means to put love before fear. To shed the skins of an identity that served a purpose but now feels false—an identity of intellect-based dominance over all that challenges us, keeping us separate from nature and our true selves. You will show the rest of us how to tap into a limitless reserve of creative energy that flows from the deepest truth of all: that we can dematerialize our egos at will and come together whenever we want.

If you are struggling, know that there is an invitation embedded in that struggle. An invitation to free yourself—your creativity—and to light your fire that feels extinguished. We all need you awake, alive, and in touch with your soul.

This very real possibility is why responding to symptoms of so-called mental illness with support rather than interference is not simply about substituting an herb for Prozac. It's about engaging in a path of personal transformation, even rebirth, so you can show up in your truest expression for what you are here on the planet to do—your purpose in this life.

---

### Resetter: Vick

I want to share a major victory I had today. I do this in the hope that someone will take heart and know that fighting for yourself is never a straight path, but that the twists and turns can serve to make us stronger.

I sang in public tonight. I haven't done that in six years. Four years ago when I was diagnosed with MDD [major depressive disorder] and severe anxiety, I had trouble even going out in public. Medication only increased my sense of dread. Singing is one of my passions, and for years I felt robbed of my ability to use that gift.

Today as it was my turn to go up to the mike, I heard all the familiar voices. The anxiety loomed. The negative thoughts said that hundreds of people would see me fail or that they would all laugh. But I found a strength that has been dormant in me for four years, a path back home to my true self.

---

## HONORING COMPLEXITY: A NEW VIEW

If we are to heal our inner artist, and free our creative spark to embody our highest self, we need a new model of ourselves as humans. That model needs to be one that honors the body as an emergent representation of the soul. Fortunately, this complexity-embracing model is being ushered in by a "new science" that reveals dynamic interconnectedness between bodily systems—the mind, emotions, and environment. This science is showing up in new fields with long names like *psychoneuroimmunology* and in a burgeoning scientific literature that explores our microbial selves.

The new science challenges the old view that if you are depressed, you were born with a brain chemical problem that you are destined to manage with prescriptions for your entire life. Instead, your symptoms are seen as representing imbalance related to lifestyle exposures that are interacting with your genes—that is, your stress, food, sleep (or lack of it), chemical exposures—and to your beliefs around the power you have to create your life. All of these variables impact how your genes are expressed and are within your control, a field of study known as *epigenetics*.

What we are learning from hard science is decimating our mechanistic perspective of the body as an input-output machine to be manipulated and managed by synthetic chemicals.

In the old, mechanistic view, the mind and body are separate, thanks in part to the legacy of 17th-century French philosopher René Descartes, who held the mind as nonphysical. The science of Isaac Newton further reduced everything of consequence to objective energy and matter: it's only real if it can be measured. Thus, modern medicine cares about observable behavior, not the deeply meaningful reason for it. In fact, patients are routinely dismissed as being "hysterical," worriers, complainers and generally less of a reliable authority on their experience than the "objective" observer. The study of the mind (invisible to the observer) is limited to the study of thoughts (rarely emotions), with an eye toward socially appropriate, productivity-oriented functionality.

Psychiatry, as a guild, has made a strong effort to legitimize itself through this lens and "make material" the mind and emotions. The problem is that perceived pathology has been reduced to the localized effects of neurochemicals, which act in a vacuum in the brain. Psychiatrists regard troublesome emotions as emerging from inborn errors of neurochemical trafficking, with a reductionist focus on the neurotransmitter *serotonin*. The mind as enemy, pumping out mood- and anxiety-producing thoughts like a ticker tape.

This view holds no consideration for the interconnectedness of immune cells and endocrine glands throughout the body or the microorganisms in, among, and around us, let alone the emerging science of quantum biology and the role of energy in our manifest experience of being.[5] Neither is there regard for the role of human emotion and its expression as an articulation of bodily imbalance, or personal suffering as a precursor for growth.

Philosopher Alan Watts, in his book *Does It Matter? Essays on Man's Relation to Materiality,* states, "According to this view, the universe is a mindless mechanism and man a sort of accidental microorganism infesting a minute globular rock that revolves about an unimportant star on the outer fringe of one of the minor galaxies."[6] He goes on to say that this "put-down" theory of humanity is extremely common among those who are still thinking of the world in terms of Newtonian mechanics and have yet to catch up with the ideas of Einstein and Bohr, Oppenheimer and Schrödinger.

I'd like to add to Watts's list another scientist, Dr. Candace Pert. Once chief of brain chemistry in the neuroscience branch at the hallowed halls of the National Institutes of Health, and author of *Molecules of Emotion: The Science Behind Mind-Body Medicine,* Pert is acknowledged as the mother of psychoneuroimmunology or *psycho-immuno-endocrinology,* as she preferred it to be called.

The implications of Pert's work are profound. Through her research and more than 200 publications in the primary literature, and in her landmark book *Molecules of Emotion,* she described the body as an information network, with the "three classic areas of neuroscience, endocrinology, and immunology, with their various organs—the brain . . . the glands, and the immune system . . . joined to each other in a bidirectional network of communication, and that the information 'carriers' are the neuropeptides."[7] In other words, our current working model of the brain is antiquated. It is not, as we have maintained, an isolated no-man's-land from which thoughts, emotions, behavior, and consciousness emerge.

Pert further asserts that the mind is in the body, and that the body is an expression of the mind, giving rise to the idea that the body's symptoms are a window into the psyche. Brain neuropeptides (strings of amino acids) travel throughout the entire body to communicate to and from the brain. Previously thought to be a hardwired network of electrical impulses, the brain, in part, conveys its perceptions to the body through peptides as the body communicates to the brain. Furthermore, the immune, endocrine, and neurochemical systems are all speaking to each other in many cellular languages, from chemical to energetic. Cells that are thought to be brain, endocrine, or immune cells all contain all of the brain and immunopeptides, creating the opportunity for trillions of communications dictated by chemical affinity for a receptor.

Our bodies are changed by the emotions we experience, and in Pert's work we have science that validates our experience. She asks us to consider the term *bodymind*, stating that our physical body is changed by the emotions we experience, that emotions are coded into these substrates that move all around the body and concentrate in "nodal points." This most certainly must be why we can change our emotions through our physical body, and also change our physical body through our emotions, further supporting the view that we can trust the body's intelligence.

Pert understood that we are in charge, never victims, stating in *Molecules of Emotion*, "Now that I know my body has wisdom, this calls for a new kind of responsibility on my part. I can no longer act like a dumb machine and wait to be fixed by the mechanic, otherwise known as the doctor. I'm both more powerful and more responsible."[8]

The field of psychoneuroimmunology (PNI) has grown from the time Pert had this insight and now has several decades of paradigm-shifting contributors. PNI acknowledges that all aspects of our physical, spiritual, and chemical bodies are connected, and disturbances to any part of the system propagate through the body. When symptoms emerge, they are meant to be a beacon; we are wired to respond to those symptoms, which are our inborn, natural recalibration system for when things go wrong. But often we respond by turning to pharmaceuticals that, according to the published literature, do more harm than good—a topic you'll learn more about in Chapter 2.

On many levels, PNI is an exciting revelation. It decimates false boundaries between different systems and allows more cohesive assessments to be made. No longer are there many blind men feeling different parts of the elephant and erroneously describing a rope and a tree trunk. We begin to see how the immune and endocrine systems appear to be in a bidirectional dialogue—a conversation between the gut and the brain. In this model, the gut influences the brain and the brain influences the gut, but they are still two separate entities communicating through biochemical signals.

This new science makes room for *you*. For your human experience that reflects deeply held beliefs, thoughts, and relationships.

One specific way PNI brings your mind and emotions into the gut-brain physiologic conversation is in the form of your stress response. But the mind is more than a response to stress; rather, it is the personal meaning of the stress that is relevant.

## ROOT CAUSES: SICK GUT, LIFESTYLE, AND PERSONAL MEANING

So if "mental illness" (including bipolar disorder, depression, ADHD, obsessive-compulsive disorder [OCD], panic disorder, and even schizophrenia) is not a genetically inherited chemical imbalance of the brain, but rather our highly attuned response to a world gone wrong, we need to look more closely at the root causes driving it. We can start by appreciating the body's language of distress—it's called inflammation. Triggered by toxic thought patterns, toxic exposures, nutritional deficiencies, and more, inflammation is a response to perceived misalignment that recruits the hormonal, immune, and neurochemical systems to participate in a new normal: an adaptation to stress.

As it has abandoned the fictitious chemical imbalance theory of depression, for the better part of the last century, psychiatric research has focused on the role of the immune system in depression, anxiety, and bipolar disorder.[9,10,11,12]

But what drives inflammation? What is it a response to? A root-cause inquiry leads us to consider at least three major categories that need to be examined for potentially reversible and resolvable contributors to the symptoms called mental illness. These are 1) physiologic imbalances, 2) psycho-emotional toxicity, and 3) spiritual crisis/emergence. There is evidence that inflammation is driven by all of these elements, and that inflammation is a catch-all alert that is adaptive if transient and symptomatic if chronic.

Let's first look at how inflammation is connected to physiologic imbalances that lead to a diagnosis of depression. If depression is a downstream collection of symptoms, and inflammation is driving these symptoms, what is a possible physical source of the inflammation? It appears, from data in animals and humans, that disruption of our gut ecology may be a major player, so the gut microbiome has stepped to the forefront of cutting-edge psychiatric research.

The other factors that drive inflammation—namely lifestyle factors such as stress from emotional toxicity in relationships and work, as well as psychospiritual responses to a suppressive society—are topics to be explored more thoroughly in Parts 2 and 3 of this book.

**Sick gut.** Our immune systems are largely housed in the gut, and the interplay between the gut and the brain is a complex and profoundly important relationship to appreciate. Housing more than 70 percent of our immune system, the gut is our interface between the outside and inside world, that separation being maintained by one cell thickness. The resident microorganisms of the gut develop into an ecosystem early in life through postnatal exposures, in the vaginal canal, through breastfeeding, and in the immediate environment, giving you your microbial template.

Disruption to the balance of bacteria through medication exposures, antigenic foods, herbicides, and stress can set the stage for the innate immune system to prepare to respond. Depression, associated with compromised integrity of this intestinal barrier,[13] emerges from the swirling storm of inflammation, impairment of vital cellular components (i.e., mitochondria), oxidative stress, and then more inflammation in a carousel-like forward rotation. Specifically, depression is associated with elevated levels of lipopolysaccharide (LPS), a component of the bacteria cell wall that is in harmony when it remains in the gut.

We all recognize that anxiety or nervousness can impact our guts; you may have had butterflies before a date or even diarrhea with extreme performance anxiety. We are just learning that this relationship is bidirectional, however, and that the gut can also communicate its state of calm or alarm to the nervous system.

Researchers posit that the vagus nerve is a primary conduit of information and that inflammatory markers are the vehicles traveling this highway. Scientists have studied the "protective effects" of severing this nerve when animals are exposed to gut-related toxins that normally cause depressive symptoms. We are getting ahead of ourselves, however, because we need to better elucidate why inflammation matters, where it comes from, and why it is the universal driver of chronic illness, including in many cases depression, anxiety, bipolar disorder, and psychosis.

**The lifestyle connection.** If we start to look at mental disorders as a multiplex of relationships between the gut and the endocrine and immune systems, as psychoneuroimmunology (PNI) shows, we begin to see how all of the threads of our day-to-day lifestyle choices weave the web of our felt experience.

After I put down my prescription pad and dedicated my practice to helping women reclaim their health—body, mind, and spirit—I found that sending a signal of safety in multiple different, simultaneous ways was all that was needed to get radical results. In effect, I operationalized psychoneuroimmunology and packaged the experience into a powerful self-care ritual that prepared patients for their journey home to themselves.

Once I started to see and then expect tectonic plate shifts in perception, symptoms, and vitality, word got out and my waiting list grew to two years. This is not rocket science, and in fact, I'm not even sure a doctor is necessary to carry it out. I wrote my first book, *A Mind of Your Own*, to lay the foundation for the journey into living an awakened life that follows in this book. Vital Mind Reset, an online program you'll read about in Chapter 6, is the exact protocol I use with my patients, informed by my own healing journey, my work with Dr. Nicholas Gonzalez, and the support of experts who will help bring this one-month experience of self-reclamation to you, anywhere in the world.

The results span from small but progressive wins to history-making cases of meds shed and disease labels defied.

One of the foundational premises of this approach is the glorious gut-brain connection, a powerful point of entry into the nervous system's wide-ranging impact on day-to-day life.

---

### Resetter: Jacie

I joined Vital Mind Reset because I've struggled with a sense of discomfort in my body and I have had a lifetime of constipation and reflux.

Since beginning VMR, I am having daily bowel movements and I can't believe how much more comfortable and confident I feel in my body. It is so clear to me that I just had to prioritize connecting to myself, taking care of myself, and give myself the chance to reset. I needed the motivation and support to finally put myself first.

---

## CINDY'S STORY: REVERSAL OF LUPUS

Cindy's story illustrates the immense power of sending this lifestyle-based signal of safety, with a focus on the gut-brain connection. Cindy was medically hexed with a lupus diagnosis after the birth of her son, and endured painful symptoms for the next 18 years. In the wake of this, and because of sociocultural conditioning around the fate of someone with this potentially serious autoimmune condition, she shrunk her life to fit what she thought the experience of a sick woman should be. She felt unwell, took multiple medications, sometimes for unknown indications, and said no to many opportunities—until she said yes and entered the realm of radical healing through diet and lifestyle changes that put her lupus symptoms into remission.

Before that, she describes her daily life: "Lupus was a drag on my system. I had good days and bad. I would get nervous about planning trips and future dates because I never knew if I would feel well enough to go. I seemed to catch everything, and had chronic sinus infections and reflux. I also had swollen, hot, and extremely painful joints most days. In the latter years, I finally figured out that food was triggering the synovitis. I just couldn't figure out which foods were causing it."

Cindy got caught up in the web of multiple medications, including a brief trial of an antidepressant. And then she heard about the Vital Mind Reset program.

Here are her own words: "I followed the protocol for 14 days, taking out foods that caused inflammation, and my body responded immediately, telling me it was food sensitivity at the root. After only two weeks, I went to my rheumatologist and had routine blood work done. When the results were in, my doctor told me that there were no signs of lupus. I nearly fell off the table! I cried happy tears all the way home, and soon received a letter from him confirming those results."

This approach to depression and other conditions views them as complex, nonspecific symptoms reflecting a state of bodily disharmony. It isn't that you were born with bad genes or low serotonin. It is far more likely that you are experiencing an unhealthy inflammatory balance, driven by cortisol dysfunction and stemming from a sick gut.

Gut *dysbiosis* (a word that translates, etymologically, to "wrong living") can stem from many lifestyle sources, including diet, environment, and stress from modern living, a topic I will cover in Parts II and III of this book.

This is where the evolutionary mismatch theory, citing modern lifestyles as the culprit, comes in: imbalanced flora in the gut due to modern diets and stress causes *permeability* of the blood/organ barrier, leading to "leaky gut" and increased levels of endotoxin (typically LPS) in the blood. Specifically, many food components have the potential to activate inflammatory responses, including modern wheat (with 15 to 20 times the gluten of ancient varieties) and processed cow dairy. Heating of foods—grilling and broiling—can also produce advanced glycation end products and heterocyclic amines. Once these dietary compounds synergize, immune thresholds are lowered as white blood cells and chemokines are readied for response.

Add to dietary influence the pharmaceutical influence, and we've engaged an all-out war on humanity. A fascinating review describes the manifold adverse effects of common medications on the gut microbiome, including anti-hypertensives, chemotherapy, and even antiretrovirals used in the setting of an HIV diagnosis.[14]

Antibiotics are, of course, notorious for their grenade-like effects, a topic we will explore in a future chapter with relevance to mental symptoms. I encourage my patients to question the use of antibiotics for this reason alone.

In summary, we need the gut lining to keep the gut contents away from the bloodstream because healthy boundaries are critical to well-being! Increases in permeability allow for intestinal contents to set off autoimmune and inflammatory processes. Because an entire inner ecosystem is in need of restoration, the solution is never going to be in a pill—natural or chemical. What's needed is the deeper healing of lifestyle change with its myriad side benefits.

## PERSONAL MEANING

With the advent of PNI, there is a new conversation happening in the medical literature: one that encompasses the whole person, all at once. However, in an article from the University of Auckland in New Zealand, researchers take the progressive field of psychoneuroimmunology to task and demand an even more nuanced and sophisticated approach to the human experience.[15] They suggest that some people will represent their meanings and "stories" clearly in language, some in behavior, some in bodily expression, and some (maybe most) in multiple ways. In this view, the "personal meaning" of one's illness is given a significant role.

I firmly believe that there is an intimate invitation in every diagnosis, and even every symptom, to examine everything from diet to spiritual beliefs. But could illness also carry *personal symbolism and meaning*? To appreciate the relevance of symbolism, the whole person must be assessed in a global view, with sensitivity to the meaning for a given individual of their symptoms.

The article's authors would agree. They propose a *co-emergent framework*, one in which mind and body are not causing effects in one another but are parts of an unbroken continuity of both internal body processes and external interpersonal meanings and influences. In other words, this is a model that takes into account the person, their story, and their environment—the whole picture.

So how can we heal on all of these levels at once: body, mind, and personal meaning? With the launch of my online self-healing program, Vital Mind Reset, referenced in the one-month protocol in Chapter 6 of this book, I witnessed that "doctor-less" healing is possible when we dismiss the reductionist, magic pill/magic bullet model and honor our web-like complexity. Medical meditation, examination of beliefs, engagement in community, detox, and nutritional medicine all synergize to bring about results that might not have otherwise been possible. When we use this multisignal, personalized (by you, for you) approach, participants marvel at the simplicity of the interventions yet the robustness of the shift.

In fact, we don't even need to know why this multilevel approach to healing works, or how. We can move beyond chemical theories and complex analysis, and simply be in the process of sending the bodymind a signal of safety.

Safety looks like ease. Trust. Curiosity. And even surrender. It's not a fight. It's not a battle. It's a cooperative exchange and an exploration. It's becoming more of our whole selves because we are becoming less fragmented and self-evasive. We stop hiding parts of our personhood from our awareness. We embrace it all, even the darkest pain, in order to heal.

CB EO

## What's Next . . .

In the next chapter, you'll learn why taking pills for your pain and suffering is the problem, not the solution, based on the latest research showing you that pharmaceutical approaches are flawed at best, and dangerous at worst.

Chapter 2

# THE PILL
# PROBLEM

*Doctors are men who prescribe medicines of which they
know little, to cure diseases of which they know less,
in human beings of whom they know nothing.*

— VOLTAIRE

In this chapter, I will take you on a tour of the research behind
the meds you've been told might save you. Chapter 2 is about how
we typically respond to pain by taking prescription medication,
why that doesn't work, and how it can even make things worse.
In order to choose how to manage your symptoms of mental and
emotional challenge, it's essential you have *true informed consent*,
and that means knowing what the science reveals about current
psychiatric practices.

**Meet Reilly**, a 42-year-old woman who is on disability and
spends most of her time at home in bed watching TV. "I've spent a
lot of my life feeling sick with no real diagnosis, but it wasn't until
my episode in college that everything went downhill," she told me.
The "episode" was precipitated by a romantic breakup and use of
alcohol and marijuana that led to several days of visual hallucinations and paranoia. Because of her long history of low mood, Reilly

was labeled with bipolar disorder and started on seven medications (yes, seven) during her first hospitalization. Since that time, she has cycled through most mood stabilizers and antipsychotics on the market and earned the new diagnosis of schizoaffective disorder. She has slowly slipped off the ledge of her formerly functional existence, has gained 60 pounds, and has few social contacts.

**Now meet Sara.** Sara lost her pregnancy weight in three weeks and felt like she could take on the world. It wasn't until she was about nine months postpartum that she felt like she'd been hit by a truck. She was sluggish and forgetful, started to gain weight and lose hair, and struggled to have a bowel movement even twice a week. She felt so overwhelmed that she knew something was wrong with her.

In a 15-minute visit, a psychiatrist assured her he knew just what that was. He told her she had postpartum depression and gave her a prescription for Paxil. Within two weeks of her first dose, she told me, she planned a suicide attempt. She drafted a letter and planned to jump out of her window. She had never experienced these feelings before, and she stated, "It just suddenly made sense. I felt calm and certain about it."

A thwarted attempt, two medication changes, and three years later, she is told that she can never live life without Lexapro and Klonopin.

Reilly and Sara are just two of millions of patients who find themselves caught in the web of psychiatric sorcery: a spell cast, hexed, potentially for life. They are told that they have chemical imbalances and the most important thing they can do for themselves is to "take their medication," which they will have to do "for life."

These patients' providers are not exploring root causes, not discussing evidence-based alternatives to medication treatment, and not disclosing the long-term risks of psychotropics, including worse functional outcomes and increased risk of relapse. Let alone the poor-integrity, industry-funded and manipulated data that supports the approval of these medications. Most egregiously, patients like Reilly and Sara are sold the false story that the medication is treating their disease rather than the truth: that the meds are simply inducing a drug effect, one that is no different from alcohol or cocaine and often as addictive.

Yet the science (hidden, archived, and otherwise ignored) clearly shows that prescribed psychiatric medications are not what we are told they are. They are chemicals that are habit forming and carry unpredictable risks, such as psychosis, suicide, and homicide. In fact, it's a game of Russian roulette: the data shows that sometimes even in the first few doses, those taking them can develop severe and irreversible adverse effects.

If you believe that depression and other mental/mood disorders are likely heritable diseases that strike at some point in a person's life, never to be undone, it makes sense that permanent medication treatment is required. But if what we are calling mental illnesses—from panic attacks to depression to psychosis—are symptoms of an evolutionary mismatch with our modern lifestyle, resulting from physiologic, psycho-emotional, and psychospiritual imbalances, such syndromes essentially invite us to revisit our day-to-day lives for the solution—not the pharmacy.

## DISCOVERY: WHY I NO LONGER PRESCRIBE

As a one-time prescribing psychiatrist, I can remember feeling like I was offering my patients a warm, nurturing hug when I gave or confirmed a diagnosis for them after a consultation. *It's the nature of bipolar disorder,* I would say. *It's part of your genetic history, a brain chemistry condition, that thankfully we can manage if you stick with your medication.* I never suspected that I was giving them cold comfort in the form of a label that reduced their human experience to an impersonal pattern so I could match it with a prescription or medical intervention.

Today, I am no longer a card-carrying pharmaceutical dispenser, although that was my training. While in college at MIT, I studied neuroscience. Then I went to medical school at Cornell University. I completed my residency and fellowship at Bellevue/NYU because I believed that psychiatrists had cracked the code of human suffering, and I wanted to do my part to alleviate pain.

I thought I was helping people when I wrote prescription after prescription throughout years of my traditional, don't-question-it kind of training. I believed that people who were struggling had a chemical imbalance and that we needed to do our best to help them access the pharmaceutical support they would need for the rest of their lives. It wasn't until I had a lived experience of radical healing that flew in the face of all of the medicine I had been taught that I went back to the books to see what other scientific evidence existed that I had not been exposed to.

In 2009, struggling with memory issues, double-booking patients and forgetting my wallet, keys, and ATM PIN, I was diagnosed with my first health problem, Hashimoto's thyroiditis, after a routine physical. An epidemic women's health issue, Hashimoto's masquerades as a psychiatric problem—anything ranging from postpartum psychosis to postpartum OCD and depression—if you don't know how to diagnosis it.

I already knew what conventional medicine had to offer: prescription drugs for life. I wanted to know if there was *another* way, so, despite my baked-in skepticism about natural medicine, I made an appointment with a naturopath. Working with her, I put my condition into remission by basically changing my diet after a lifetime of eating cheese and bread every day (I was raised Italian-American!). My naturopath was an academically oriented woman who didn't waft sage in the corner, and I began to see that, unlike what I'd been brainwashed to believe about such approaches during my pharmaceutically funded training, her alternative approach was evidence based. Within months of dietary change, I saw my thyroid antibodies move into normal range, and I was convinced.

I began to look deeper at the research regarding prescription medication. What I found out was shocking. I learned that in an effort to help, doctors prescribe medications that move symptoms around in what looks like a game of whack-a-mole. When a drug suppresses or distorts a symptom, it doesn't actually resolve, and that disturbed energy manifests elsewhere, often in a more complex and disabling set of symptoms. So as patients are falling off cliffs, psychiatrists are offering them knives to grab on to, help that ends up making them sicker, or at best arresting an emergent and self-limiting process.

This is the perspective of several renegade psychiatrists and of Robert Whitaker, whistleblower, investigative journalist, and author. His book *Anatomy of an Epidemic* reported non–industry funded literature that I hadn't been taught about in my education and training, and reading it changed my life. In 2010, I put down my prescription pad for good, and I have not started a patient on a single medication since.

Through further research in non–industry published literature, I learned how psychiatric medication can perpetuate the very disability that it purports to resolve. In other words, you are worse off taking it than not. Hard to believe, I know, because we feel like we have to do *something*, and medication is what we typically do in urgent and serious situations. You'd be reckless or stupid not to avail yourself of the safe and effective tools Western medicine has to offer—and perhaps even combine it with some Eastern methodologies for the best of both worlds, right?

If I needed to dive deeply into the research to learn this, how could the non-clinician—especially *you,* the consumer—ever expect to be accurately informed?

Obviously, it was the right timing and the gift of my illness that allowed my mind to open to new possibilities. For starters, I had personally put into remission a potentially debilitating chronic disease—a remission that my training taught was not a possibility, let alone a goal. Because I was awakened to a broader version of the body's innate healing capacity, and because I was learning that long-term medication outcomes were abysmal, I began to offer my patients the opportunity to come off their medications and finally address the root cause of their original symptoms. More on what that looks like, soon . . .

## THE LIE WE'VE BEEN TOLD

"All I know is that Prozac saved my best friend's life," said an agitated young woman sitting in the third row of the conference room during the Q&A of a lecture I'd just given.

I field this sentiment often and remember feeling the resistance myself when I began to confront some of the data that undermined what I had been taught about the safety and efficacy of psychiatric medications. After all, we've been told that these meds are:

- An antidote to brain chemical imbalances
- More effective than placebo
- Safe for everyone, from babies to the elderly
- Recommended for long-term use
- Non–habit forming

But the truth is that many market forces and industry interests have shaped your belief that medications like antidepressants and anti-anxiety medications are safe and effective. The literature tells a different story, namely that this "treatment" approach can, in fact, lead you down a path of chronic illness and multiple new diagnoses. No one actually wants to take medications for life. No one believes that health comes through a prescription bottle. But we feel backed up against a wall, and when we are offered a way out, of course we take it.

The real snake oil salesmen of our time are those offering you this quick fix, entirely undermined by available evidence, without a word of the real risks and the deeply meaningful, inexpensive, and effective alternatives. If you are informed of the risks, benefits, and alternatives to a given treatment, you will be empowered to make the best decision for yourself based on your personal, family, philosophical, and religious life context. But the truth is that prescribers are not in a position to share the known risks of medications because they learn only of their purported benefits, along with a short tagline about dismissively rare risks that are thought to be invariably outweighed by the presenting clinical concern.

But in order to choose, you have to know what's possible. This is perhaps the most important truth I have to share, one that is predicated on a principal tenet of ethical medicine: *informed consent.* Informed consent implies the exploration and confirmed awareness of all known risks, benefits, and alternatives. In addition to peeking behind the curtain of medication efficacy and safety to see the small man pulling the strings, you need to know what is really possible in order to make a choice that feels empowering to you.

For example, did you know that you can put schizophrenia, bipolar disorder, OCD, panic attacks, chronic fatigue, ADHD, major depression with suicidality, eating disorders, and generalized anxiety into total remission without medication, and even in spite of it? Did you know that you can shed these labels and walk into the wilderness of your life only to encounter the real you?

But if you *don't* know what awaits you on the other end of your dance with medication, you might imagine that euthanasia[1] or suicide are the only options. My mission is to make sure that as many people on this planet as possible know that the presumed "incurability" of chronic disease is a myth and that healing is eminently feasible, because only *then* can you truly make an informed choice.

Unfortunately, the medical system is not set up to provide informed consent any more than a butcher is set up to discuss the benefits of veganism. Even the most serious risks, including impulsive suicide and homicide, are minimized as rare and random. The FDA and the pharmaceutical industry have gone to great lengths to conceal multiple signals of harm, so you certainly can't expect your average prescriber to have done the investigative work required to get at the truth.

In fact, from 1999 to 2013, psychiatric medication prescriptions increased by a whopping 117 percent, concurrent with a 240 percent increase in death rates from these medications, according to U.S. Department of Health and Human Services survey.[2]

According to data gathered since in the U.S. National Health and Nutrition Examination Survey, about 37 million Americans are prescribed antidepressants (13 percent of the population), and half of those prescriptions are of at least five years in duration.[3] Adults over 45, women, and whites are more likely to take antidepressants than younger adults, men, and minorities. But usage is increasing in older adults across the demographic spectrum.[4]

White women over 45 account for about one-fifth of the adult population but account for 41 percent of antidepressant users, up from about 30 percent in 2000, the analysis found. Older white women account for 58 percent of those on antidepressants long term. The number of long-term users seems to be piling up year after year.

No one is safe, not even children: 7 percent of boys and 5 percent of girls are medicated with psychotropics;[5] 10,000 toddlers under three are prescribed stimulants,[6] and there has been an 8,000 percent increase in children and teens (0 to 19) treated for bipolar disorder.[7]

## THE INDUSTRY AND THE MARKETPLACE

So what's driving the seemingly ill-informed and irresponsible dispensing of these drugs to the public on such a large scale? To answer that, we need to look at what's going on in the world of big business where the decisions are made to produce and market the drugs you are promised will help you. Surprisingly, the science and the profit-making world are more than in bed together; they are in a long-term relationship that is currently flagrant in its disregard of the damage inflicted on the general public.

But this isn't some kind of conspiracy in which malevolent people sit in a room and plot to harm people. This is the way the system works. It's an alignment of politics, profits, and incentives. We have a system that richly rewards people who prioritize commercial applications for drug research. And this system is, itself, a symptom of our quick-fix consciousness that has lost connection with meaning, beauty, and the sacred. We are asking for the quick fix, and thus, new drugs are fast-tracked through the approval process. Inconvenient risks—short term and long term—are ignored, and many important questions about the impact of these drugs are left unanswered. A lot of what we really need to know to have the more complete story about medications is locked in a drug company's file drawer cabinet.[8]

In fact, only two "adequate and well-controlled" studies are required for FDA licensure of pharmaceuticals, essentially leaving the population to participate in a post-marketing experiment in which adverse effects—causalities—are monitored passively.

Most prescriptions for antidepressants are doled out by family doctors, not psychiatrists, with 7 percent of all visits to a primary care doctor ending with an antidepressant prescription.[9] Furthermore, it's been shown that most people who take antidepressants never meet the medical criteria for a diagnosis of major depression, and many who are given antidepressants for conditions like OCD, panic disorder, social phobia, and anxiety also don't qualify as having these conditions, even according to the questionable criteria that the *Diagnostic and Statistical Manual of Mental Disorders* (*DSM*) itself puts forth. In one study, researchers determined that "among antidepressant users, 69% never met criteria for major depressive disorder (MDD); and 38% never met criteria for MDD, obsessive-compulsive disorder, panic disorder, social phobia, or generalized anxiety disorder in their lifetime."[10]

*Do the best you can until you know better.*
*Then when you know better, do better.*

— MAYA ANGELOU

## WHAT THE SCIENCE SAYS

Let's review some of the evidence suggesting that it may not be in your best interest—or in the best interest of those around you—for you to travel the path of medication-based psychiatry. Making those choices in a fuller landscape of available information gives you a better chance of engaging in *informed consent*.

Here's my list of the top four reasons—logical, intelligent, evidence based—you don't want to get on the antidepressant treadmill:

- They are ineffective, often resulting in worse long-term outcomes than no treatment at all.
- They can unpredictably induce psychosis and violence toward self and others.
- They are habit forming, even addictive, and discontinuing them may entail excruciating withdrawal.
- They are unnecessary; there are other ways, with robust side benefits.

I'll unpack the science and rationale behind each of these, but first I want to report the shocking truth I learned from my independent research about psychiatric medications: *there is no valid scientific basis for their use.* The truth is that in seven decades, not a single human study supports the idea that depression is caused by a certain kind of chemical imbalance in the brain. Imaging studies, postmortem suicide assessments, and animal models have never yielded consistent patterns of brain chemical levels, metabolites, or receptor profiles.

So if there's no science behind them, how did antidepressants become so universally accepted and prescribed?

As I reported in my book *A Mind of Your Own*, the predominant theory behind modern antidepressants (SSRIs, or selective serotonin reuptake inhibitors) is that they work by increasing the availability of serotonin, a neurotransmitter famously associated with mood. In fact, if you were to quiz someone on the street about the biology of depression, they would likely parrot "chemical imbalance" in the brain and go so far as to say a "serotonin deficiency." This hypothesis is referred to as the *monoamine hypothesis*, and it grew primarily out of observations made in the 1950s and '60s.

This idea that these medications correct an imbalance that has something to do with a brain chemical has been so universally accepted that no one bothers to question it. But the truth is that *the serotonin theory of depression is a total myth* that has been unjustly supported by the manipulation of data.

The brain is much more complex than the serotonin model can describe. To be clear, SSRIs cause an overstimulation of serotonin receptors, making them less sensitive over time, a process called *downregulation*. This explains the documented phenomenon of antidepressant *tachyphylaxis*, the loss of antidepressant efficacy over time,[11] and *tardive dysphoria*, a worsening of the original symptoms continuing for a period of time after the discontinuation of the medicine,[12] as well as the incredible strain on the nervous system during withdrawal. In the first 12 years after its initial marketing debut, Prozac was named in more than 40,000 reports of adverse effects submitted to the FDA.[13] No other drug on the market comes close to such a history.

So now we must ask: Just how effective, really, are the drugs so many are prescribed for depression? What are the short- and long-term effects? Are they addictive? Can they cause violence to self or others? And are they necessary, or can basic lifestyle interventions facilitate the body's powerful self-healing mechanisms to end depression?

Let's let the science reveal answers to these questions, starting with psychiatric drug effectiveness.

## Effectiveness: Failure to Deliver

A recent study led by Irving Kirsch, now associate director of the Program in Placebo Studies at Harvard Medical School, reanalyzes primary outcome data from the Sequenced Treatment Alternatives to Relieve Depression (STAR*D) study.[14] The STAR*D was the largest, longest, and most expensive study ever conducted to evaluate depression treatment. It sought to establish "real world" conditions, assessing and tracking outpatients who were treated for all sorts of coexisting medical conditions (as in real life) and without randomization to placebo. Results of Kirsch's reanalysis study suggest inflation of antidepressant efficacy (specifically, in patients taking citalopram) both in the STAR*D trial reports and in conventional clinical trials. Of note, at the end of the one year STAR*D trial, only 3 percent of the original subjects maintained remission.[15]

Importantly, the STAR*D trial lacked a placebo arm to help us understand how much of the analyzed effect might have been attributable to the passage of time or belief, the latter of which, Dr. Kirsch has demonstrated, is a major driver of psychiatric outcomes. In 1998 he published a meta-analysis of 3,000 patients who were treated with antidepressants, psychotherapy, placebo, or no treatment.[16] He found that only 25 percent of the therapeutic response was attributable to the drug's action. This was followed up by a 2008 review, which invoked the Freedom of Information Act to obtain access to unpublished studies showing that when these were included, antidepressants outperformed placebo in only 20 of 46 trials (fewer than half!).[17] Kirsch refers to the "active placebo effect" as the potential for known drug "side" effects (dry mouth, constipation, headache) to be perceived as evidence that the study participant is receiving the active medication rather than placebo, therefore breaking blind. This is further corroborated by data that shows no separation from placebo when an active placebo is used (aka a medication like atropine with similar "side effects"). Thus, believing that you are being treated leads to the outcome of perceived improvement.[18]

There are many examples in the medical literature of the power of mind to influence the body. A Harvard study took 84 hotel attendants with cleaning responsibilities and told half of them that their daily work satisfied the surgeon general's recommendation for exercise as part of an active lifestyle.[19] They told the other half nothing. The group that believed their activities satisfied the surgeon general's recommendations showed a decrease in weight, blood pressure, body fat, waist-to-hip ratio, and body mass index. The stunning conclusion of the study: *"These results support the hypothesis that exercise affects health in part or in whole via the placebo effect."* Then there are the patients at UC Davis undergoing spinal surgery who had 45 percent less blood loss when they practiced a brief pre-surgical visualization technique.[20]

This is powerful stuff. Add to these studies the work of the brilliant author and scientist Bruce Lipton, aimed at awakening us to the reality of our beliefs and their influence on the expression of our genes, a factor that may be the most important determiner of our health and wellness. In his popular YouTube lecture, Dr. Lipton says, "The placebo effect should be the subject of major, funded research efforts. If medical researchers could figure out how to leverage the placebo effect, they would hand doctors an efficient, energy-based, side-effect-free tool to treat disease."[21]

So why do antidepressants "work" for some people but not for others? A recent study attempts to answer that question by exploring the biology of the placebo effect.[22] Researchers used brain scans to determine who was most likely to have an exaggerated response to 10 weeks of antidepressant treatment. They determined that those who had more opiate receptor sites (tiny "doorways" on the surface of cells that give access to pain-killing substances, both natural and pharmaceutical) open and available were more likely to respond to an "active placebo" (they were told it was a highly effective and fast-acting antidepressant), and also more likely to experience relief with a subsequent antidepressant. Interestingly, this effect was more active in women.

In an effort to acknowledge the legitimacy of this phenomenon, a *New England Journal of Medicine* report attempts to explain a physical mechanism for the placebo effect, involving activity in the brain: "Placebo effects rely on complex neurobiologic mechanisms involving neurotransmitters (e.g., endorphins, cannabinoids, and dopamine) and activation of specific, quantifiable, and relevant areas of the brain (e.g., prefrontal cortex, anterior insula, rostral anterior cingulate cortex, and amygdala in placebo analgesia)."[23]

It seems that the dismissive expression *it's all in your mind* might better be rephrased *it's all in your brain* to be closer to the truth.

## Long-Term Losses

You might find yourself asking, So if they work, even if because of the placebo effect, who cares? It's better than nothing, right?

Wrong. In fact, not a single long-term study demonstrates (remember to read beyond the reported outcome!) that you would be better off taking medication than if you hadn't at all (or discontinued shortly after starting). In fact, this is the premise of intrepid journalist Robert Whitaker's work and educational efforts: to boldly share inconveniently suppressed data, telling a story of physician-caused harm through chronic psychotropic exposure.[24]

Whitaker posits that the negative outcomes are related to "oppositional tolerance," or the way in which the body adapts to these chemical exposures, leading to a new (and less healthy) normal rather than resolving an underlying imbalance. He invokes the Hippocratic oath, stating that in order for a medication to do no harm, it must result in better outcomes than the natural course of illness. He argues, using non–industry funded literature, that medications have turned what might have been a single episode of depression, mania, or psychosis into a chronic, recidivistic disability.

We have to dig into the archives to learn what the natural course of any of these symptoms might look like, however. For example, he cites a study funded by the National Institute of Mental Health entitled "The naturalistic course of unipolar major depression in the absence of somatic therapy" to illustrate that 85 percent of depression resolves spontaneously in one year without intervention relative to the 15 percent or less we can expect through medication as evidenced by the true analysis of the STAR*D.[25] And this does not even take into account the injury incurred by the 23 patients who will be labeled with new-onset bipolar disorder because their antidepressant medication effects are categorized as symptoms of a new illness.[26]

The long-term outcomes are the same for bipolar disorder, anxiety disorders, and treatment of ADHD with stimulants where the results of the often misreported study of stimulant use in children actually conclude, "At the end of 36 months, medication use was a significant marker not of beneficial outcome, but of deterioration. That is, participants using medication in the 24-to-36-month period actually showed increased symptomatology during that interval relative to those not taking medication." Medicated children were also slightly smaller, and had higher delinquency scores."[27]

You might be tempted to assume that those diagnosed with schizophrenia obviously need medication and would do worse without it. Whitaker reports on a seminal study by Martin Harrow that found that at the end of 15 years, 40 percent of the schizophrenia patients who had stopped taking antipsychotics were recovered, versus 5 percent of those who had stayed on the drugs.[28] This was followed by a seven-year randomized study published by Wunderink in the Netherlands that corroborated the above outcome.[29]

Our impression that there is a single psychiatric diagnosis that is better off medicated in the long term comes from a carefully crafted marketing agenda resulting from industry influence on prescribers. Whitaker has single-handedly exposed that the literature has long since indicted the use of these medications as perilous for patients in need of a different kind of support.

## Adverse, Even Dangerous Side Effects

"It feels like I'm plugged into an electric socket and every move I make shoots voltage throughout my body," a patient interested in tapering off medication reported recently. "I'm nauseous and my stomach feels like it's on fire. Of course, I can't sleep, and I spend the whole day thinking something terrible is happening. I have to tell you, there's no way I can live like this."

This patient's experience is not uncommon. Adverse physical side effects of psychotropic drugs commonly include:

- Agitation, shakiness, anxiety
- Flu-like symptoms
- Indigestion and stomachaches
- Diarrhea or constipation
- Loss of appetite
- Dizziness, disorientation, confusion
- Insomnia or sleepiness
- Headaches
- Low sex drive, erectile dysfunction, difficulties achieving orgasm
- Weight gain
- Excessive sweating
- Heart rhythm problems
- Muscle twitching or pain
- Shivering

When reporting these effects, patients are often told to "hang in there," that these kinds of problems generally improve with time. But when they don't resolve, doctors start tweaking. They'll adjust the dose or add a second and a third medication. What they typically won't tell you is that things can veer dramatically off course, and more dangerous side effects are possible.

Pharmaceutical companies typically list side effect risks for their drugs, but we can't rely on those reports, which minimize what people actually experience. A current study of the adverse effects directly surveyed an international sample of antidepressant users. They were asked whether they had experienced specific adverse effects as a result of taking the antidepressant, and if so, to what degree of severity.

The responses came from 1,431 people in 38 countries. Results showed 61 percent of the respondents reported at least half of the listed adverse effects, most commonly: feeling emotionally numb (71 percent), feeling foggy or detached (70 percent), feeling not like myself (66 percent), sexual difficulties (66 percent), drowsiness (63 percent), and reduction in positive feelings (60 percent). Suicidality was reported by 50 percent, withdrawal effects were reported by 59 percent, and addiction by 40 percent. One-third did not recall being told about any side effects by the prescriber. Fewer than 5 percent were told about suicidality, emotional numbing, withdrawal effects, or addiction.

What this study shows is that when we ask people directly, rather than relying on reports from pharmaceutical companies, far higher rates of adverse responses to antidepressants are revealed than were previously known, especially in the emotional, psychological, and interpersonal domains. The report concludes, "Given recent findings that antidepressants are only marginally more effective than placebo, the findings of this study imply a cost-benefit analysis that cannot justify the extremely high prescription rates for these drugs."[30]

## Violence-Inducing Effects

You may not know that antidepressants have a well-established history of inducing violent-behavior side effects, including suicide and homicide in previously nonsuicidal, nonviolent people. In fact, five of the top ten most violence-inducing drugs have been found to be antidepressants.[31]

It's even possible that antidepressants can cause a sane person to act like a cold-blooded criminal.

On an unseasonably chilly day at King's College in London, I arrived to give a two-day workshop to clinicians and laypeople interested in mental health. I was there to share what I have learned about the medications that I so dutifully and faithfully prescribed during the early part of my career, and about the potential for healing depression in simple, safe ways, according to the latest science.

The day before my flight, I had received an e-mail from a man whom I would choose to invite onstage with me that day. He wrote, "I took the life of my 11-year-old son Ian on July 31, 2004 in a Paxil-induced state of psychosis and was charged with first degree murder. I was judged to be 'not criminally responsible on account of a mental disorder' in September 2005 and received an absolute discharge from the forensic psychiatric system [in Ontario, Canada] in December 2009. I've been off all prescription drugs since September 2010. Prior to our family tragedy, I was a physically active sports consultant with no history of violence or mental illness."

He told an audience of clinicians and patients that day about how it is that a common citizen, prescribed a seemingly safe medication for work-related stress, goes on to commit a heinous act of violence against his beloved child. This academic classroom was heaving with grief when he finished his description of events.

Individuals perpetrating unspeakable acts of impulsive violence against self and others are not a new phenomenon. What is new is the altered states of consciousness induced by antidepressants and other psychotropic drugs that are well documented as promoting homicidal and suicidal behavior in susceptible individuals. This, in addition to other factors such as loss of social connection, loads the gun and pulls the trigger.

There is an untold story of the vast and irreversible risks of psychotropic drugs doled out to millions without any rigorous diagnostic procedure, any screening for risk vulnerabilities, or any true informed consent about what is known about the amplified benefits and the suppressed risks of these interventions.

A 2011 study examined ten patients with variants in a drug-metabolizing liver enzyme who committed homicide (primarily of children and family members) after being started on psychiatric medications. They returned to their baseline personalities after medication discontinuation, highlighting the intoxication effects of these chemicals.[32] *Just one* of these cases should have led to the ban of the entire class of medications. Unfortunately, not much has been done with this information and you probably haven't heard a whisper about this particular paper.

You may not know that there is also a database at ssristories.org and another called murdermeds.com maintained by intrepid activist Andrew Thibault (a father who sued the FDA for hiding evidence of the violence-inducing potential of stimulants, and won), where these media-making cases of psychotropic-induced violence and impulsivity are documented, including school shootings, kamikaze plane crashes, and infanticide.

More recently, 17 students and adults were killed in the Marjory Stoneman Douglas High School shooting in Parkland, Florida, by 19-year-old Nikolas Cruz. An investigation by a state agency concluded that Cruz was taking medication for attention deficit hyperactivity disorder. The most commonly prescribed drugs for ADHD are methylphenidate and amphetamines, which combined spell *methamphetamine*, commonly known on the street as "speed." Such stimulant drugs given for ADHD are considered controlled substances, similar to methamphetamine and cocaine.

You might think this is rare, and that these people are "mentally ill," so obviously they are on medication.

The truth is that pharmaceutical companies have been working overtime to suppress a signal of harm around violence with these psychiatric medications—coding negative outcomes in short-term trials as "emotional lability," punting those cases to the placebo group, and otherwise discounting impulsive violence that populates the treatment arms of drug trials.

It's time to start taking these medications seriously and seeing them for the brain- and body-altering chemicals they are. Until we know more about whose life might be irreversibly and irrevocably altered by even a single dose of psychiatric medication, we must honor the physician's oath to *first do no harm*. This means asking *why* a patient is struggling, and entering with support and lifestyle changes that can offer relief within days to weeks—all without a single side effect.

## Suicide

If you've read recent reports that state "U.S. suicide rates surge to a 30-year high," you might make the connection that things feel very *wrong* in our world today. This is the report of the National Center for Health Statistics, showing increases in every age group except older adults.[33] The rise was particularly steep for women ages 45 to 64, jumping 63 percent over the period of the study; for men the rise was 43 percent in that age range, the sharpest increase for males of any age. These increases lifted the nation's suicide rate to 13 per 100,000 people, the highest since 1986—documenting the "30-year surge."

For reasons that remain mysterious, those under the influence of psychiatric medication often specifically choose to hang themselves in their moment of peak impulsivity. Kim's husband, Woody, who was never depressed a day in his life but was prescribed Zoloft by his internist, even verbalized a felt experience of his head coming apart from his body in the days before he was found hanged in his garage.[34]

Then there's 14-year-old Naika, a foster child in Florida who hanged herself on a Facebook livestream after being treated with 50 mg of Vyvanse, a drug treatment for ADHD that leads to a domino effect of diagnoses and psychiatric meds, including a thirteen-fold increase in the likelihood of being prescribed an antipsychotic medication and a four-fold increase in antidepressant medications over controls.[35]

Are these just rare anecdotes? Is this just the cost of treatment that is helpful for most? Are we blaming medication for what might have been severe mental illness that was undertreated and/or undiagnosed?

There's no denying it: on a personal, national, and planetary level, people are suffering to survive, and the distress is coming from all sides—medical to economic to existential. You may find yourself in agreement with seemingly logical appeals to provide these individuals more help and greater access to treatment. But that may be

43

the last thing our population of hopeless and helpless needs. Life's inevitable challenges are not the problem. It's the drugs we use that are fueling the rising rate of suicide.

Over the past decade, I've learned through my research into the literature that the data tells a very different story about the safety of psychiatric medications. In general, there are two characteristically distinct groups of individuals who commit suicide: those who have never been in psychiatric treatment, and those who have. According to available data—three large meta-analyses—more psychiatry means more suicide.[36],[37],[38] In multi-country, large-scale longitudinal studies, suicide rates have increased while at the same time we've increased psychiatric funding, treatment, and access.

How could this be? As many prominent voices including Robert Whitaker, Dr. David Healy, Dr. Peter Gotzsche, Dr. Peter Breggin, Dr. Irving Kirsch, and Dr. Joanna Moncrieff have researched, the untold story of psychiatric medications includes their propensity to induce violence, in otherwise nonviolent individuals, against self and others. This is a shocking assertion: the medications we are offering to help those in distress may be leading patients to the very outcomes we are most hoping to avoid.

Prescribed specifically to "prevent" suicide, antidepressants have come with a black box warning label of suicide risk since 2004. Multibillion-dollar lawsuits have been necessary to unlock the cabinet drawers of an industry that cares more about profit than human lives. In fact, based on his research, Dr. Peter Gotzsche, founder of the Nordic Cochrane Collaboration, who was recently removed from its leadership because of his pharmaceutically critical research, claims, "Our citizens would be far better off if we removed all the psychotropic drugs from the market, as doctors are unable to handle them. It is inescapable that their availability creates more harm than good."[39]

## Addiction: Creating a Monster

Here's a dirty little secret in psychiatry: Starting meds can be easy, but stopping—not so much. In fact, I've come to the conclusion that psychotropic medications—from Lamictal to Ativan to Effexor and everything in between—are the most habit-forming chemicals. On. The. Planet. Crack cocaine, oxycontin, and alcohol don't hold a candle to the physiologic withdrawal that even a slow taper from these medications can induce. Before I developed the one-month Reset protocol you'll read about in Chapter 6, I was running an out-patient rehab center for withdrawal-induced disability that made my patients look like they were suffering from acute-onset AIDS. Full-body pain, rashes, hair loss, menstrual abnormalities, electric shocks, racing heart, stomach bleeding, and more. And that's not to mention intractable insomnia, loss of appetite, intense terror, cognitive impairment, and impulsive agitation.

Patients are told that reduction schedules vary based on the drug, the dose, the duration, and previous symptoms. It sounds scientific enough. But the truth is that coming off antidepressants can be a horror show, and not a single physician in America is trained in how to safely discontinue these medications because the need to do so is just beginning to be acknowledged. In fact, it wasn't until 2014 that the medical literature even began to reflect that psychotropic withdrawal was a distinct medical entity. In the first systematized review of SSRI withdrawal, researchers examined 23 studies and 38 case reports, which led them to conclude that the euphemistic term "discontinuation syndrome" must be abandoned in lieu of a more accurate depiction of the habit-forming qualities of antidepressants: withdrawal.[40] Yes, just like Xanax, Valium, alcohol, and heroin.

According to an article in a Harvard Medical School publication, "There are no hard and fast rules for getting off antidepressants . . . some can taper off . . . in a matter of weeks, while others may take months."[41] I would even add *years* to that statement based on a 2018 U.K. report that analyzed 24 studies to create a more accurate portrait of the experience of withdrawal. It reveals that antidepressants are far more addictive and harmful than was previously assumed.

Highlights from the paper are as follows:

- More than half (56 percent) of people who attempt to come off antidepressants experience withdrawal effects.

- Nearly half (46 percent) of people experiencing withdrawal effects describe them as severe.

- Sixty-four percent of patients say their doctors never warned them about the risks or side effects of antidepressants.

- It is not uncommon for the withdrawal effects to last for several weeks or months.

- Current U.K. and U.S. guidelines underestimate the severity and duration of antidepressant withdrawal, with significant clinical implications.[42]

The main purpose of the study was to examine the severity and duration of antidepressant withdrawal effects, and whether or not the official U.S. and U.K. warnings given to patients were sufficient, telling them that effects are "self-limiting (typically resolving between 1 and 2 weeks)" and "usually mild," according to American Psychiatric Association guidelines as well as the fifth edition of the *Diagnostic and Statistical Manual of Mental Disorders* (*DSM-5*).

But researchers revealed a very different picture. "Current clinical guidelines are in urgent need of correction," noted study researchers John Read, a psychologist, and James Davies, a cultural anthropologist. "While in some people, such reactions may be mild, of short duration and manageable . . . in other people . . . these reactions are severe, long-lasting, and can make normal functioning impossible. Typical AD [anti-depressant] withdrawal reactions include increased anxiety, flulike symptoms, insomnia, nausea, imbalance, sensory disturbances, and hyperarousal. Dizziness, electric shock–like sensations, brain zaps, diarrhea, headaches, muscle spasms and tremors, agitation, hallucinations, confusion, malaise, sweating and irritability are also reported," along with "mania and hypomania," "emotional blunting and an inability to cry," and "long-term or even permanent sexual dysfunction."

What this should tell you is: A) the people establishing the guidelines don't really know, and B) it might not go so well. All you have to do is spend a few minutes on survivingantidepressants.org, beyondmeds.com, madinamerica.com, or ssristories.org to appreciate that we have created a monster. Millions of men, women, and children the world over are suffering complicated withdrawal symptoms routinely dismissed by their prescribing clinicians.

Contrary to what the pharmaceutical industry would have you believe, weaning off psychotropic medications can be extremely difficult. While there are no official numbers on how many people are attempting to wean themselves off their drugs, a recent study of 1,829 users of antidepressants found that about 75 percent had tried, just over 30 percent of them quitting successfully; the others found the withdrawal symptoms too hard to bear.[43] Choosing to take these drugs could mean signing up for a serious rehabilitation process if you choose to discontinue them later in life.

## JAYNE'S STORY: BENZODIAZEPINE DEPENDENCY

A 63-year-old librarian, Jayne came to me six months into her process of tapering from the benzodiazepine Klonopin, a drug prescribed for anxiety. She had long ago abandoned her original prescriber—the one who put her on Remeron and Klonopin eight years ago after she discovered her husband's infidelity.

"My doctor never once told me there might be an issue with taking these meds long term," she reported. "In fact, he told me I probably still needed them after I tried stopping cold turkey and felt so sick I thought I was dying."

When she arrived in my office, she had been using a jeweler's scale to measure micrograms of shaved Klonopin tabs to approximate 1 to 2 percent dose decrements per month. She told me of a hell that she had never envisioned possible before her tenure in the world of psychiatry.

I have countless stories like Jayne's from my work with patients dependent on psychiatric medications. There are a reported 100 million prescriptions for benzodiazepines written annually, with long-term prescriptions written for 14.7 percent of 18- to 35-year-olds and 31.4 percent of 65- to 80-year-olds, and with women twice as likely to be prescribed.[44]

How did we get here? People started on one, maybe two medications, that turned into three, maybe five medications over years of their lives during which they never felt fully well and may have even struggled just to function. *Just a little more of this medication . . . maybe this new one will help* . . . No one ever discussed with them the risks, benefits, and alternatives, simply because we as clinicians are not exposed to the full story . . . unless we seek it out ourselves.

As an intern working in Bellevue Hospital's intensive care unit, I treated a patient who presented after having suffered a grand mal seizure in the CVS parking lot on the way to fill his Xanax prescription. He had missed one dose before heading to the store. After that, I never prescribed Xanax again, but reassured myself that Klonopin and Ativan were safe because of longer half-lives and slower onset. Now I suffer the poetic justice of caring for dozens of patients who are moving through the birth canal of Klonopin withdrawal, and I am here to guard the gates through which more may pass.

Xanax, Klonopin, Ativan, and Valium seem to spell simple relief. Unfortunately, there is no magic pill, and no free lunch. Whether antidepressants, mood stabilizers, antipsychotics, or benzos, they all bring you to the same room. It's a room that many spend years trying to escape. It's one of dependency, depression, forgetfulness, and detachment from self, all states that have been catalogued by Dr. Peter Breggin in his books dedicated to documenting the nervous system–injuring potential of these medications. The science is there; it's simply time to accept it and to do better by those in need of support and healing.

## ANOTHER WAY

In sum, the science behind these drugs' outcomes, both short term and long term, presents a dismal picture of their capacity to really help you heal, let alone even effectively manage or suppress the symptoms that are overwhelming you. On review, there's no good case to be made for their effectiveness, they have dangerous side effects potentially leading to homicide and suicide, and they are extremely difficult to withdraw from. This failure of the medication route is what leads patients to my door, where they are asking, *Isn't there another way?*

The laundry list of acute and chronic adverse effects is growing, and the unpredictable risk of medication-induced violence should lead to an urgent cessation of all psychotropic prescribing. We live in a cultural context that makes no room for the relevance, meaning, or significance of symptoms. Symptoms are simply bad and scary and must be managed. We must begin to make room for patients to ask *why* they are not well.

If all this isn't enough to convince you that taking psychotropic medication is not a good idea, consider an even more compelling reason, one that is the theme of this book: prescription medication robs you of the opportunity to understand why you were symptomatic in the first place. It's a Band-Aid, and a not very helpful one at that. Considering that the drug's effectiveness is only on the level of placebo, and taking into account all of the risks (harmful long-term effects, dependency, violence-inducing behavior), the *Why?* inquiry should start to sound more worth the effort.

So what does this mean for you? It means this: If you are taking a medication, it is still worth getting to the root cause of why you needed one in the first place. And if you're considering taking medication, I recommend that you read Chapter 6 and consider first committing yourself to my one-month protocol.

If you knew that your symptoms were reversible, healable, and transformable, you might consider walking a different path instead of assuming the level of risk you are undertaking in exchange for the placebo-level efficacy of psychotropic medication. In fact, every person I have ever tapered off psychiatric drugs into total vitality once believed that they would have to be a medicated psychiatric patient for life. If you knew that radical self-healing potential lies within each and every one of us, if you only knew that was possible, you might start *that* journey today. It's side-effect free.

## Travel Tips

To support you along the way, I'll be offering Travel Tips, summarizing and even introducing some important points for your journey.

I'm including two "quick win" tips for the start of your journey beyond suppressing symptoms with drugs, showing you how small interventions can shift your emotional state within minutes to hours. The result is that you can feel into a very different story about yourself and your body's ability to naturally recalibrate.

### Tip #1: Change Your Breakfast

Are you eating cereal, bagels, muffins, or other quick fixes for breakfast? Are you feeling like you need a coffee drip flowing through an IV? Are you hungry and irritable about an hour and a half after breakfast? Treat yourself to some body-hacking and see how you feel with a different breakfast. Balancing blood sugar to impact mood can be as simple as increasing natural fats in your diet.

People often ask me what I eat for breakfast. If you're looking for a quick and easy recipe to improve brain health and functioning, and give you energy to spare, try my KB Smoothie. Loaded with healthy fats, lecithin, protein, and antioxidants, this smoothie packs a serious punch—and it tastes great![45]

Here's the recipe:

- ½ cup frozen organic cherries or berries
- 8 ounces fermented coconut water, coconut water, or filtered water
- 3 tablespoons collagen hydrolysate as a protein base
- 1 tablespoon sprouted nut butter
- 3 pastured egg yolks
- 1 tablespoon coconut oil
- 1 to 2 tablespoons ghee
- 1 to 2 tablespoons raw cocoa powder

Blend and drink!

## Tip #2: Calming Breath Meditation

When fear is driving you to reach for the quick fix, try this simple breathing meditation that is associated with calming and cooling. Start with practicing it 3 minutes a day.

- Sit in a cross-legged pose.
- Close your right nostril with your right thumb, while your other fingers are stretched straight up as antennas. Your left hand is on your left knee.
- Close your eyes and concentrate at a point between your eyes and slightly higher (the yogic "third eye").
- Begin to breathe long and deep only through your left nostril.
- Continue for 3 minutes.

## Tip #3: Mental Floss

When I trained at the Bellevue Hospital in New York, where there were 14 locked inpatient units, the outpatient psychiatric center was marked by a sign that said "Mental Hygiene Clinic." I think of this seemingly anachronistic phrase often, and smile to myself about the hidden depth of that awkward phrase. Today, mental hygiene seems to be the mandate on the path toward self-discovery: clean up your mind. This means generating an awareness of your thoughts and electing to give attention to only those thoughts that represent your creative power, aka who you want to be. Observe your thoughts all day, and treat them like guests coming to be seated at your beloved restaurant. Do you like their vibe? Or do you think it's better to pass on them? You have the power to give them a table or tell them, *I'm sorry, we are fully booked at the moment. Have a nice evening!*

Focus on thoughts that make a statement of *who you really are*. Otherwise, lean away and think again. Take control of the energy of your thoughts so you can lean into your emotions instead, and explore the experience of them without immediately attaching a story to the feeling.

C33 80

## What's Next . . .

In the next chapter, we explore how there is a purpose to our pain, and how, when we start to inquire about what that purpose is, we can begin to truly heal.

Chapter 3

# THE POINT
# OF PAIN

*The foundation of all mental illness is the unwillingness
to experience legitimate suffering.*

— C. G. Jung

Can you remember the last time you really just let it hurt? The
last time the burning in your chest felt like it was going to pull you
into the molten center of the earth? The panicked disorientation—
the simultaneous desire to explode, implode, and run away? Do you
remember what you did with that pain, sadness, anger, hopelessness? Did you eat differently, drink differently? Did you hide from
it? Did you work more? Did you vent its intensity as irritability and
lash out at someone? Maybe your own child? Did you reach for some
form of medication, whether a prescription or not?

We don't like pain—any kind of pain, be it a headache or heartache—ours or really anyone else's. We avoid it at all costs. The trend
in our culture is to pathologize any kind of suffering, to make it
a problem, a disease, an emergency, and to numb, suppress, and
silence it. After all, in the West, we are allowed the modest goal of
*managing symptoms* and are almost never told we can reclaim our
vitality *through* them. The consequences of this management are
that we don't get to grow, don't get to follow what the canary in the

coal mine is telling us to do, which is to look at our lives and our world and act from that bigger picture.

In this chapter, we will look at how pain and suffering serve an important purpose, one we can understand as a pathway to healing and transformation, physically, emotionally, and spiritually.

## PATHOLOGIZING PAIN

Ancestral cultures have long appreciated the role of desperation, struggle, and breakdown in transcending the existential crises that inevitably befall every human in their lifespan. It's called *initiation*. From Africans to Australian aborigines to Native Americans, men are initiated through injection with poisonous frogs, wearing gloves filled with stinging bullet ants, wilderness survival, psychedelic plants, tooth removal, and even ingestion of their own foreskin without chewing. Movement through the fear and pain induced by these planned, anticipated, and culturally supported processes allows participants to touch their inner refuge of strength, trust, and surrender.

Women in tribal cultures have their own rituals when they transition from girlhood to womanhood, almost all of which involve singing and dancing. And of course, all women have built into the design of their being the potential for the greatest initiation: childbirth.

We, as a culture, reject these initiatory rituals. In fact, we are enculturated to prize keeping it all together, even if what we are keeping together is a false, unfulfilling life experience and we are inadvertently preserving an adolescent consciousness well into our adulthood. When we are confronted by life experiences that seem too painful, too demanding, or too overwhelming to bear, we are supported in running from them, avoiding them, or otherwise shrinking back into our familiar normal. These experiences, however, are opportunities that may very well serve as rites of passage. We prize comfort above all else, imagining that it actually exists. We suppress and distract ourselves from the messages that keep coming: the invitations to step into our adult power.

We forget that tears—emotional tears—heal. In fact, when you let yourself cry, you release prolactin, adrenocorticotropic hormone (ACTH), and leucine-enkephalin, none of which are secreted when you cut an onion. Our bodies are built to dance with this connection to ourselves, to feel pain, accept it, and let it open us bigger to receive more joy.

But in our modern psychiatric/medical paradigm, the unfortunate trend is to pathologize suffering and other challenging emotions. Distress is a sign of sickness to be eliminated by consciousness-suppressing drugs, not a gateway to change. It is not an invitation to look at what might be misaligned or out of balance. Instead, we are driven by fear to engage a system that makes us sick and then offers us chemical cures that beget more chemical cures. We are told not to trust our instincts, not to consult our heritage for models of wellness, never to honor the inner wisdom of our bodily organism over the seemingly exacting mechanism of modern science.

But if pain serves a role in our well-being, what happens when we try to numb, silence, or become desensitized to it? And how have we come to a place where we go so far as to call *crying* a symptom of illness? Weeping, sobbing, wailing are perhaps the most human expressions of all; in fact, we are the only species on this planet that cries. Seems like it might actually be an essential expression to honor, no?

It used to be that someone going through a bereavement could *not* be diagnosed with a major depressive disorder. But since 2013 that exclusion has been eliminated. With the fifth edition of psychiatry's diagnostic manual, the *DSM*, there has been a "lifting" of the bereavement clause. This means that even if you have just suffered a trauma or the death of a loved one, you can be diagnosed with *major depressive disorder*, the gold standard treatment of which is an SSRI antidepressant. You only need to be struggling with five out of the following nine symptoms to get that label:

1. Low mood
2. Loss of interest
3. Decreased appetite
4. Changes in sleep
5. Changes in activity
6. Fatigue
7. Feelings of guilt/worthlessness
8. Poor concentration
9. Suicidality/hopelessness

Imagine experiencing a profound loss, like the death of a loved one, and instead of being supported to deal with your grief, you're told you have a medical problem in the form of major depression and should start taking mind-altering drugs. Or what about welcoming the birth of a child into the world, and suddenly you're a little more anxious than before, sleep-deprived and fatigued? What if that anxiety is a wise response to the fact that you, a new mother, are spending much of your time alone, without a tribe of other women around you supporting you and teaching you how to enter this new phase? How can that be called an anxiety disorder that needs to be medicated? It only can if the context of these symptoms is not taken into consideration, not deemed as critical.

What are the consequences of this tendency to relegate our sadness and grief to labels and then try to suppress them? Where do the sadness and grief go if we bandage our awareness of them with overwork, medication, addictive substances, or a general avoidance of our real human experience? They get buried and we don't feel our own feelings, the good as well as the bad. We become numb, and the numbness feels worse than pain because our hearts will always remind us when they are closed. This is why disconnection represents a struggle far more chronically trying than the fire of any initiatory pain, grief, sadness, or fear, fully felt.

## SORROW AND GRIEF: A RUGGED TERRAIN

Perhaps you feel as I once did, that grief and sorrow are feelings to be avoided that may only have a rightful place in the setting of death and loss. If you haven't experienced a recent death or loss, grief and sorrow probably aren't a part of your healthy life experience, right?

As a tough Type A'er, before I learned how to make room for feelings and to flow in my life rather than manage it (which involved shifting my priorities toward pleasure and self-care, tolerating the attendant fear of loss of income and productivity), I never allowed myself to experience the bubbling up of intense emotions like sadness, grief, and despair. If I felt a twinge, it would almost instantly get translated into irritability because of how overwhelming it can be to manage to-dos and feel at the same time. The feeling was still there, but because I didn't make room for it, I now had to get back to business as usual, with a good portion of my attention diverted to keeping the volcano suppressed. However, as my well-controlled and manicured lifescape began to rupture, I came into contact with immense subterranean sadness and sorrow. Exploring them has allowed me to live larger, to expand emotionally, and to heal dysfunctional patterns driven by unacknowledged fear and pain that were keeping me stuck and small.

It was during this time of encountering my own painful emotions that I was ready to pick up Francis Weller's book *The Wild Edge of Sorrow*, a primer on all of the sadness that comes along with simply being human.

As explored in Chapter 1, we have strayed from evolutionary alignment, and our bodies, minds, and souls are rebelling in service of our awakening. But we don't know this, and we think of that rebellion as annoying and tedious, a sign we are broken and not able to conform to expected standards of appropriate behavior. We are told that it's normal to go through life feeling a pervasive sense of not-okayness, and that if it begins to interfere with "functioning," and shoring up on coffee, sugar, shopping, and workaholism isn't cutting it, there is a pill that could help.

In his book, Weller writes:

> When we abandoned the Old Ways, established over hundreds of generations, we lost the traditions that made us feel held and embodied. The psychological, emotional, and cultural design that offered us assurance and security in the face of grief or loss has been replaced by a belief system that generates anxiety and a sense of insecurity. Emptiness now saturates our culture. Addictions, consumption, and materialism are symptoms of this condition. More accurately, they are attempts to cope with the unbearable feelings of barrenness.[1]

Weller implores us to appreciate the fact that all people before us knew the power of communal ritual in processing, discharging, and transforming these layers of grief, including death and loss, trauma and shame, divorce from nature, isolation from community, and the ancestral pain we inherit through *morphic resonance* when information is passed down (and around) without actually being encoded genetically. (Morphic resonance is a concept described by scientist Rupert Sheldrake in his book *Morphic Resonance: The Nature of Formative Causation.*)

One of Weller's "gateways of pain" we must pass through that struck me was our isolation from community, something I have felt the absence of as if it were a phantom limb. We used to wake up to many eyes every morning. Now we are raising children as single parents, living in modular homes, and privatizing our rightful pain and struggle.

I remember, after my second daughter was born at home, attending a Red Tent meeting and sitting in a circle with about 20 strangers. A Red Tent is a gathering of women that occurs at the new moon for girls and women most in need of support, rest, and reflection. It recreates a timeless tradition observed by ancient cultures and serves as a contemporary forum for empowering women's sense of selfhood. We sat in a circle and told our stories of our birth experiences. Most of the women there had experienced redemptive home births after in-hospital traumas, but I'd had two transformative and empowering experiences and little to grieve, or so I thought.

Nonetheless, from the start to the finish, I wept. I wept so intensely that I couldn't even share my story. I didn't even know that I had wanted this—these compassionate ears and hearts sitting with me, open and real. A renegade and a mercenary, I'd always had an *I can do it on my own, I don't need anyone* kind of posture toward life. But now I understand that a deep, oozing wound inside me was the absence of a tribe. Every time I am in community, I heal a bit, I open a bit, and I shed something dysfunctional that was compensating for that pain.

## THE SOURCE OF OUR PAIN: CHILDHOOD TRAUMA, WOUNDING, AND PROGRAMMING

I want to add an additional kind of suffering we endure and must heal to become fully human: the traumatic impact of the emotional and psychological wounds we incur in our childhood.

In my private practice, nearly 100 percent of the women I work with identify as having experienced childhood trauma: verbal, physical, or sexual abuse and/or domestic violence. The perceived injuries range from a mother's critical reaction to a math test score in first grade all the way to heinous and ongoing sexual violation. Trauma expert Dr. Bessel van der Kolk, author of the important book *The Body Keeps the Score*, writes, "Trauma causes people to remain stuck in interpreting the present in light of an unchanging past."[2]

Thus, repeated patterns of perceived victimization arise, perhaps to show us, like a persistent tap on the door of our soul, that this pain *requires healing*. Our reflexive response to these patterns is often referred to as *reactivity*, as in re-act, or acting again from a past imprint rather than to the context of present life experience, and defines the places, people, and things that hold the power we need to reclaim in order to heal. In fact, anything that gets you hot under the collar is probably tripping a trauma wire, firing off programs of felt abandonment, betrayal, inadequacy, and shame. Such programs have stories attached to them that keep us feeling a surrogate sense of control because at least we are *right about being wronged*. Our entire personality gets cozy with the familiarity of these *poor me* emotional patterns, choosing to attract and enact them again and again.

We go out of our way to co-create experiences that confirm our beliefs, and especially the core belief most of us carry—*I'm not enough*—or its sibling variant, *I'm too much*. For example, I have a programmed belief that no one has my back, that when things get tough, no one can or wants to be there for me. They can't handle me and everything I am, and I will be abandoned because of it. I developed this belief through a childhood wound, and for many years of my life I collected experiences that confirmed that belief. I would find that colleagues scattered when I came under media attack, that family and friends abandoned me in one of my Dark Nights, or that I repeatedly failed when trying to assemble groups of like-minded researchers and clinicians. It took uncovering the source of these experiences, taking responsibility for my childhood wounds, and approaching life with increased self-awareness and open-hearted vulnerability, an ongoing process, for me to begin to heal and stop attracting these kinds of situations.

In ways, we are all still operating from our internal "child-self" (a term I use to point to childhood pain), focused on striving toward the good (love) and running from the bad (withdrawal of love) because we got the message, at some point in our upbringing, that the good was welcome and the bad was, well, bad. As we run from the bad, however, we abandon the part of ourselves that needs reclamation in order for an experience of wholeness, relegating it to the shadows. It is that part of ourselves that we have been taught by society, our parents, and our internalized inner critic to hate. That shameful, lazy, weak, stupid, ugly loser inside each and every one of us.

I tell my patients that it is as if we have locked our childself in a bedroom, bolted the door, and turned up the music loud so that we don't have to hear her wailing and banging. Then we arrange the furniture just right, dust the house, and wonder why it just doesn't seem to feel quite like home. In that bedroom is your neglected childself, begging to be unconditionally loved, to finally feel seen, heard, and safe. If denied, that child will continue to tantrum in order to get your attention. Those tantrums look like self-sabotage, depression, anxiety, and the emptiness of a life based on arranging externalities.

Because we are walking around as man-boys and woman-girls, unaware of our inner pain and the associated defenses, we project this so-called shadow material onto the bad person, the bad genes, the bad germ, or the bad luck that is responsible for our suffering, rather than seeing our lived experience as a reflection of our relationship to ourselves. We are no longer ceremonially initiated by our tribespeople to confront our inmost terrain in order to become adult men and women, so we are all still being driven by our childhood programs set in place to protect us from the pain of rejection, abandonment, and betrayal.

For example, my parents are very good, kind people, and yet I developed two prominent programs in response to challenges in childhood that I call The Mercenary Program, aka I can take care of myself on my own (a response to feeling inadequately loved, protected, and supported) and The Lighthouse, aka I will be forever scanning for problems I can fix and focus on so that I am never caught being wrong or responsible for a bad thing (a response to feeling loved conditionally for my good behavior). If I am aware of these reflexive aspects of my personality, I can mine for and choose to explore the strong emotion beneath.

We carry these unprocessed and avoided emotions in our bodies, and our bodies try to show us that we can run but we can't hide. The suppressed emotions, when they erupt, are called *symptoms*, *illness*, and *disease*. It is in this way that an internal child runs our lives until we turn toward her, acknowledge her, honor her needs, feel her feelings, and translate her truth through our loving, self-possessed, and clear adult consciousness. Always beneath the surface, this wounding program is activated by anything and everything that smells like, feels like, looks like, or behaves like the characters from our primary injury. The wound wants to be seen, and so it is always actively commanding our attention, but identifying with it as a disease (*I'm a cancer patient* or *I have depression*) is like saying that the smoke alarm is the reason the house is burning down.

Facing your wounding from childhood and working with the relationships that will help your childself feel heard is the hardest work you will be asked to do in a lifetime. It is the work that breaks familial cycles of disempowerment and sets you, and the rest of us, free. The work begins by acknowledging that there's somewhere you have not wanted to look. There's some primal fear that you've been running from your whole life. There's something big you have to forgive, a conversation you know deep down you have to have, a heavy secret you've been towing around. That house of cards that you've held up for decades might need to fall. The confusion, pain, and disorientation that can come with that will characterize you reaching your rock bottom. Rock bottom is when you can run no more. It's when it's time to turn, face your shadow, and bow down in surrender.[3]

---

### Resetter: Shay

During my daily meditation practice I have started to take out a photo of myself at age 6 to try and send her love and let her speak. And OW OW OUCH is it painful to see myself there, so young so innocent so pure so hopeful and so unaware of what was coming down the tracks. And I'm seeing that I can't hate her, loathe her, punish her, hide her away, judge her, shame her, and I'm recognizing that she is me. It's confronting, it's uncomfortable, it's maddening, it's painful, it's difficult not to look away from her. But she's screaming for me to look at her, so I am.

---

## FIGHT, FLIGHT, OR FREEZE

Trauma leaves an enduring mark not just on our beliefs, our psychology, and our emotions, but principally on our nervous system.

One day, while we were walking from his office toward the subway in Manhattan, my mentor, Dr. Nicholas Gonzalez, turned to me and said, "You know what the top five most important contributors to health are?" I dug deep, listing off inflammation, the microbiome, the role of nutrients, until I realized that this was a question my previous training in functional medicine likely hadn't prepared me to answer. He said, "The autonomic nervous system, the autonomic nervous system, the autonomic nervous system, the autonomic nervous system, and the autonomic nervous system." He literally said it five times, counting out each utterance on his fingers. He was referring to the nervous system that controls our glandular secretions, our heart rate, and everything "automatic" about our being that also assesses and orchestrates responses to any state of alarm in the body.

At the intersection of neuroscience, evolutionary biology, and psychology, research scientist Dr. Stephen Porges contributed the polyvagal theory,[4] which adds important nuance to our understanding of the autonomic nervous system. He describes how, going beyond that system's functions for rest/digest and fight/flight, the vagus nerve, often conceived of as simply a parasympathetic rest-and-digest conduit between visceral organs and the brain, has evolved many different hierarchical roles.

Porges describes the vagus as having two branches: a more ancient, unmyelinated branch below the diaphragm, responsible for reptilian-like freeze (and defecate) responses called the *dorsal vagal complex*; and a relatively newer branch above the diaphragm that lowers heart rate and controls facial expressions and vocal tone, called the *ventral vagal complex,* or the "social nervous system."

In times of safety, this vagal system supports rest, digestion, and regeneration; however, in times of perceived danger, this system mounts the more ancient defenses of dissociation or fainting, including dizziness, nausea, and intense fatigue. The social nervous system allows us to recruit a sense of safety from others and the environment, and to pair sympathetic activity with play (think lively dancing), or immobility with peace (think deep meditation). What Porges calls *neuroception,* or how our nervous system assesses the safety of settings and people, can be influenced by trauma and conditioned responses and beliefs.

For example, if you were assaulted by someone in a red jacket, the sight of a red jacket in your periphery can set off a sympathetic fight or flight, or even a parasympathetic freeze in the setting of sufficient danger perception. If we are able to establish that the environment is safe, however, and to glean from cues like facial expression and voice prosody that an individual means us well, this higher-functioning social network role of the vagus nerve suppresses our more primitive fight/flight and freeze responses. This state of vagal tone also allows us to remain calm and present when faced with another's suffering, enabling experiences of compassion or bearing caring witness as a means of activating the sending of safety signals between us.

Do you ever feel more anxious when you try meditating? In those with trauma histories, engaging in exercises designed to induce calm (such as breathwork) without a sufficient sense of safety in the setting can induce vulnerability, because for these people, calm can be associated with lack of vigilance and subsequent danger. Those who experience agitation when attempting to meditate, for example, are likely undergoing activation of their fight/flight system in response to induction of calm through active contemplative practices. This is a response that would be adaptive if the threat were, in fact, ongoing, which is essentially what our nervous systems perceive in states of chronic traumatic impact.

For these individuals and others, the parasympathetic system can be supported and toned, and body awareness enhanced, to allow for more conscious engagement with the environment and life experiences. Toning of the parasympathetic through breathing (including lengthened exhales), chanting, and bowing postures can allow our vagus to remain online to balance out perceived danger with a dampened defensive response. This vagal tone also facilitates compassion so we can support another in their moment of struggle without getting sucked into a vortex of pain. Much of what is explored in this book will serve to repair and heal this imbalance.

*How can I be substantial if I do not cast a shadow?*
*I must have a dark side also, if I am to be whole.*

— C. G. JUNG

One participant in my Reset program shares how she faced her pain to end a vicious cycle of chronic pain, depression, and physical disability.

## LEANNE'S STORY: FROM PAIN TO MEANING

Before starting the Vital Mind Reset program, Leanne was crippled with full-body pain and deep depression that had kept her a prisoner in her house for most of seven years. She was 37 when it hit, pregnant with her third child, and in an unhappy marriage, surviving an unfulfilling life as wife, mother, and homemaker.

She tells of how she suffered from trying to stay positive and do everything right. "I spent seven years in tortuous hell. Unbearable physical pain, shame, guilt, anger, fear, unworthiness swirling around like a black hole devouring all in its path, panic attacks that lasted for days. I was unable to function and could barely even walk."

In the Reset program, Leanne got the message of her pain: "I've been dismantling all that for these past 18 months, realizing that my pain was the manifestation of years of unhappiness and anger over having given up my career and trying to be the perfect mother and wife. But now I've tipped the scales in my favor. I've been waking up with joy and love in my heart, and peace. I've released years of anger and emotional pain that started in my childhood, and learned to love others because I have learned to love myself. I forgive myself and no longer punish myself."

With her new mental and spiritual mindset, Leanne faced her fears of not being able to work. She called her old boss and got her job back, put her kids in school (no longer home schooling), and started a new life. "I know now I was ready to embark on my journey. I'm still on it and will be my whole life. There is no destination—I don't need to be anywhere but where I am each day."

On the program's Facebook group, she posted: "We're all in this together, even though it is different for each one. I was hopeless. I was lost forever in darkness, but, really, I wasn't. Neither are you—you only think you are." (You can find Leanne's story on the Video Testimonials tab on my website.)

You cannot avoid this step of facing your wounding on your way to reclaiming your true self. There's a term for attempts to skip over this important stage, called "spiritual bypassing," when you might be tempted to move on to "higher states" while overlooking and ignoring the cries of the inner childself who lies helpless in the dungeon of your psyche. Having the courage to embrace that wounded child leads to the energetic shrinking of your parents and childhood authorities, so they become a smaller part of your psychic landscape. Like Dorothy did in *The Wizard of Oz*, you must look behind the curtain to see the small man pulling the levers to operate the illusion.

Through this process, you re-parent yourself, your childself within, through the development of witness consciousness and a clear separation and individuation from that feeling, sensitive child within. Only then will you lessen the frustrated need of your childself to be seen and honored. Ideally, at this point, you are held by others in your community who authentically see you and honor you, because we aren't meant to do this work alone.

## SITTING WITH THE PAIN: SURRENDER

Pain is a powerful captor. In your life, you may have known heartache and loss, and it feels like you are suffocating. You want to scream and explode as much as you want to fade into nothing. It twists inside you and threatens to rupture your vital organs. You hold your heart as it bleeds, knowing that if you squeeze it too tight, it will stop beating, and if you let it go and walk away, you will die.

Fear goads. It demands and begs you to act. *Fix it, you idiot!* your fear screams. Fear tells you the lies it must in order to get you to move. *You are going to feel like this forever. You've lost everything you needed. This pain you're feeling is something you deserve. Life from now on is suffering. Nothing matters anymore.*

You try to negotiate. To be still and go through, not around, is excruciating beyond measure. To accept what is being delivered—to accept what *is*—feels like the hardest thing you've ever done.

But why should you even bother? Why permit yourself to have a painful experience? What's the point?

We sit with pain because it is how we finally surrender and enter the crucible for our transformation. This is where and how we evolve. It's how we learn. It's how we shed skins to become new.

Surrender can only come when you let go and give up control. It is not giving up, walking away, saying *forget it.* Surrender is letting go of control so you can feel into the design of it all, knowing it is not your design. In fact, it may never look the way you thought it would. Surrender lets you zoom out and take it all in, feeling held by the grandeur of the larger universe as your micro-world falls apart.

With perspective, you'll see your experience of sitting with pain as a test of faith, a true exploration of how much you are willing to relinquish the illusion of control over your path, how much you understand that the unfoldment is only to be witnessed, not managed, and that the people and things you lose are what you needed to shed in order to stop living a lie. But it's the hardest thing to do because the mind must be quieted for this to happen. We have to say *shhhh* . . . over and over again. We have to find that silence in order to let go.

When I sit with pain, I know that it is transforming me inside. It is refining and reconfiguring and upgrading all that needs that. What emerges will be closer to truth, more resilient, and more real, even if I don't like it at first. This pain doesn't need to be understood or narrated. It just needs to do its work with my consciousness, allowing it by holding space for it in order to honor it.

The thing is, we don't know how to do this. We've lost touch with it, and no one teaches us anymore. We don't even know that it's an option to consciously confront our hurt, fear, rage, and inner wildness. And that's why we feel stuck, detached, confused, overwhelmed. We walk through life asleep because we have constructed an entire existence around avoiding pain and discomfort. As Michael Singer depicts in *The Untethered Soul*, we build an entire robotic apparatus around a splinter in our arm so we don't aggravate it. But there is a way to take it out and heal it. We are buying into the fantasy that avoiding pain is even possible. As a result, the pain becomes a chronic, dull, existential ache instead. We try to ease it with medication, with drugs, with sex, with work. We do everything we can to keep it all from falling apart, as if protecting this familiar world is the most important agenda.

Yet that is what we need to do, let it fall apart, in order to be transformed.

## YOU ARE THE WOUNDED HEALER

My daughter loves Harry Potter (and so do I). In his early training as a wizard, Harry is learning to cast an advanced protection spell, and in order to make the spell work, he must conjure a powerful feeling of happiness. He can only connect to *one* moment, however, in his life that he would have ever characterized as happy. In the story that follows, we learn that Harry is a deeply traumatized character who translates his wound, through his increasing intimacy with inner pain, into an understanding of the good object and bad object in every person. He understands that his inner darkness is a part of the alchemical mixture that allows him to experience his own gifts.

Harry's hero's journey is yours as well. You are learning to wield and use your darkness, your pain, and to bring your magic to the world and to others. This is the path of the wounded healer.

In fact, it may be the case that your perceived and labeled "brokenness" is the exact place where your greatest and most powerful gift lies. Your emotions, your distractedness, the ways in which your soul says yes or no to different relationships and life experiences, are all reflections of your immense energetic power—a power that requires mastery to wield. Through this lens, the defining crisis point in your life is your emergence, your initiation, the beginning of your acceptance of your gift and the road toward your most embodied power. This self-discovery is the discovery of the mystery and perfection within and without, and it is only possible when you turn toward your wound and gather up your entire self.

It makes sense that this bigness of energy within you is terrifying—not only to others, but to you. It makes sense that you would develop elaborate defense mechanisms in an attempt to control your life and make yourself small to meet conformist expectations. It would make sense that you would be apt to misuse this power, and to give it away to a system that calls it "illness."

It is in the reclamation, however, that you develop intimacy with it and knowledge of its nature, and you can direct it in the service of healing, helping, and supporting others struggling to connect with higher channels of energy and with themselves. You learn to align your desires, thoughts, speech, and actions into a creative force: a force that empowers you to make the seemingly impossible possible for yourself and for the collective. When you heal, you make it more possible for others to heal, not only directly, but indirectly, through your energetic contribution to the field of possibility.

## TRANSFORMING PAIN

On a Thursday morning, I'm in a Kundalini Yoga class with my teacher and dear friend, Swaranpal. After some brief warm-ups, we begin a set of what she calls "rebirthing *kriyas*," exercises that are particularly powerful. We start with our arms out in front, hands clasped and index fingers extended, and then rotate from the shoulders in a circular motion. "We are carving a hole in our subconscious," she says and laughs. "And our subconscious is eight minutes thick."

Having a teacher-training certification in Kundalini Yoga, I know how to relate to the discomfort that is fast arising in my shoulders, probably only one minute into the exercise. I know that pain reaches a ceiling, and then it lingers there for a while, even though my mind tells me it could keep on getting worse forever. I know that the pain, at some point, will transform into a tingling sensation, and if I commit to it, if I just choose to continue, then something interesting might happen.

In this case, the something interesting is an emotional release. As my body shakes and my mind screams, I persist. Soon the pain turns into a sensation, and as this happens, tears start flowing down my face. Not of joy, not of sorrow, just of aliveness. Of beingness. Of release of what is no longer needed. And then comes the integration, the bliss of putting my arms down and letting it all swirl inside. I call this experience the *wave of life*, a metaphor for how our encounter with pain shifts and changes with time, moving through our experience like water.

In this and in so many ways, suffering—letting yourself feel your pain—is meaningful. To find that meaning in every single experience that comes your way, receiving and engaging with curiosity at the same time, is your ticket to freedom. In fact, this is the fundamental difference between medicated consciousness and medicine-less consciousness. Let go of the mandate to resist and fight everything and anything that feels outside of your control, and play with the idea of saying, *I don't know, but I'm sure there's something in here for me.* This is the way out of your victim story.

Psychiatry wants you to live in a meaningless world and dismissively calls this process of meaning-making "referential thinking." But the emergence of the new science and quantum physics, along with the consciousness movement, shows you that you can break out of the cage you are in. You can do it, and all it takes is a curious perspective on your hardship, and the belief that your journey is in the service of your highest expression.

Your pain is your greatest teacher, and suffering is an opportunity to evolve into yourself more fully. There are no exceptions. Miscarriages, deaths, affairs, and losses of all kinds can leave you a hapless victim reaching for a quick fix to ease the pain, or these experiences can carry you to higher ground.

When you let yourself feel your pain and get curious about its meaning, you transform yourself to become:

- **Authentic.** Authenticity: you can smell it, sense it, and detect it. When you have dipped into the depths of your own shadow, you present to others as someone who is real, not someone scrambling to guard hidden wounds. You can be trusted and depended on.

- **Empowered.** Exploring your suffering and going through the process of integration and alignment mean looking under all the rocks, clearing the cobwebs, and exploring the blind spots. When you do this, you develop an invincible core because vulnerability is a part of your strength. You have all you need to meet any and every challenge.

- **Alive.** You can feel all of it: the full spectrum of emotions from bliss and ecstasy to the electric richness of a heart scorched by pain's lightning strike. Don't accept a gauze-wrapped existence.

- **Present.** When you have sorrow that you refuse to set a space at the table for, you are constantly managing that suppression, part of your attention always preoccupied with hiding. You become susceptible to the illusion that you can create a safe life for yourself through your external trappings. You live in the future as you run from the past. But if you allow for it all, you release all of the energy that was going toward making everything okay, and that energy is free to propel you into the present moment and your real-time experience.

- **United.** When you sit with sadness, grief, and pain, you make it that much easier for others to do the same. When you accept the love and support of your fellow humans, you offer them the gift of compassion, through which they and you are healed. You can't do this life alone, especially hiding in a bunker of your own distorted story of unexamined suffering and shame, dressed up and masquerading as medicalized mental illness.

---

### Resetter: Misty

I understand more clearly now that depression is a meaningful symptom of a biological mismatch with lifestyle. . . . Because of this program, I am in the process of choosing, beginning *my* new story, engaging in *my* radical transformation, and saying yes to a different life experience. I couldn't hear my heart all these years: I didn't know there was a song for my life in another key. Thank you from the bottom of my now singing heart!

---

You may not have access to spiritual midwives the way I have had, and the way I provide for participants like Misty who take my program, so you must learn how to first be that midwife for yourself—to tell yourself this very simple message, over and over again, like a mantra: *Just. Let. It. Hurt.*

## REBIRTH: ACTIVATING YOUR INNER FORCE

One of my teachers, the intuitive holistic healer and spiritual mentor Joseph Aldo, shared this tale in a workshop to help us appreciate the power of a natural process when witnessed rather than interfered with.[5]

A man found a cocoon of a butterfly. One day a small opening appeared. He sat and watched the butterfly for several hours as it struggled to force its body through that little hole. Then it seemed to stop making any progress. It appeared as if it had gotten as far as it could, and it could go no further. So the man decided to help the butterfly. He took a pair of scissors and snipped off the remaining bit of the cocoon.

The butterfly then emerged easily. But it had a swollen body and small, shriveled wings.

The man continued to watch the butterfly because he expected that, at any moment, the wings would enlarge and expand to be able to support the body, which would contract in time. Neither happened! In fact, the butterfly spent the rest of its life crawling around with a swollen body and shriveled wings. It never was able to fly.

What the man, in his kindness and haste, did not understand was that the restricting cocoon and the struggle required for the butterfly to get through the tiny opening were Nature's way of forcing fluid from the body of the butterfly into its wings so that it would be ready for flight once it achieved its freedom from the cocoon.

The implicit message so often transmitted to patients by psychiatric medication treatment is *Hurry up and get it together and get back to your routine.* Is life really about hurrying up? Any more than dancing is about moving from point A to point B? When you prioritize markers of productivity and achievement over the richness of your journey, your essence is sacrificed. There is no shortcut to birthing your true self: learning about the emotions you've been running from and the story they want to tell, and transforming that fear into the love you didn't think was there or could ever be felt. This is an inside job that involves the shedding of your false self you thought the world wanted and the birth of the rarified you the world truly needs you to be.

## YOUR INITIATION

If you are in the hole of pain, here's what I have to say to you: This is your initiation into your greater self, your transformed and awakened self. Are you ready for your initiation? Do you want to move into a freer, more actualized version of yourself, to get closer to the unconditional love you haven't yet even experienced, and to know better what it is that you are here to do, not from your ego but from your soul?

To do that you must move through the birth canal of your process and into the light. Be humble. Look for a way to try on a different perspective and a new approach to struggle that honors it rather than rejects and laments it. It's here whether you like it or not, so work with what you can take from it. Can you be more gentle? Can you commit more fully? What about being right? Can you let go of that? Do you need to connect more fully to your tribe, to yourself, to carry you through the next challenge?

When I struggle, I reach back inside myself to the births of my daughters. I visit with the experiential knowing that it is always darkest before the dawn. I remember the feeling of white-hot fear and deep inadequacy induced by a physical sensation so intense that I thought it might kill me. *I don't think I can do this. What if I just can't do this?* I remember negotiating and seeking reassurance from my homebirth midwife. I doubted myself a thousand times, and most in the minute right before my daughter was born, and I was remade inside myself. I was chiseled to reveal more of who I truly am as a woman. I met with my inner infinity and my connectedness to the whole. For the rest of my life, I will draw from that knowing.

We all need to come together to create space for these transformations. We need to honor each other's processes and to witness and allow rather than meddle and correct. Every time you move through your own personal fire, you make it more possible for someone else to do the same. This may be the deepest way to weave us back together into the fabric that will hold us through any and every eventuality.

*You have come here to work out an individual plan for*
*your own salvation. . . . You are saving yourself*
*from the oblivion of non-realization.*
*You cannot lose in this battle. You cannot fail. Thus it*
*is not a battle at all, but simply a process. Yet if you do*
*not know this, you will see it as a constant struggle.*

— NEALE DONALD WALSCH

## ALI'S STORY: FROM DISABILITY TO REBIRTH

My office was Ali's last stop. She and her family were looking for residential facilities because her symptoms were so disabling, chronic, and unresponsive to conventional treatment. She had collected diagnoses over her lifetime including eating disorder, premenstrual dysphoria, depression, generalized anxiety, and bipolar disorder. She had made five real suicide attempts, had been hospitalized multiple times, and was delusionally agitated for several days around her period every month.

What unfolded in two months defies everything I learned in my conventional training. We implemented the steps I outline in my book *A Mind of Your Own* and the online Vital Mind Reset program and tapered her off medication, and she was not only symptom free, but reborn.

"Never in my wildest dreams did I think that even ten years ago I could have the peace that I am experiencing in my life as I am now," she told me. "Not only am I alive, I *feel* alive. I want to be alive. I am one hundred percent following the diet, doing coffee enemas once a day (two a day around my period), practicing Kundalini every morning at 4:30 A.M., and talking to [my EFT practitioner] twice a week. I am engaging with the world, no longer getting 'hooked' by triggers and negative energy. I am still healing but realize how powerful and strong I am to have survived what I did."

Ali's case is now published in a peer-reviewed, indexed journal.[6] You can see the video of my interview with her on my website, on the Video Testimonials tab.

## Travel Tips

As you take the path of surrender rather than resistance, no longer dismissing or masking your pain and suffering, you will find your curiosity takes you deeper and deeper into an inquiry about the source. This journey is not for the weak of heart. You'll need all the help you can get.

### Travel Tip #1: Become Aware

When you are struggling, when you feel pain, or even when you feel overly excited or activated, simply note it. Label it. I am angry. I am scared. I am frustrated. I am sad. Healing starts with this awareness, so bring it to as many moments of your day as possible, but don't necessarily translate it into some ambitious fix.

1. Feel discomfort.
2. Pause and note the discomfort.
3. Label it with an emotion: anger, sadness, jealousy, shame, pain.

That's it! Sounds simple, huh? It's the hardest, but most critical first step to self-authority and mastery.

### Travel Tip #2: Have Self-Compassion

This is not the same as making excuses for yourself, babying yourself, or lowering the bar. This is about understanding the tenderness that motivates your stuck behavior, your rigidity, your negativity. It's about looking beneath your habits of control and self-criticism and your layers of victimization, and learning more about the hurt that these behaviors are trying to protect you from.

Beam love and soul-acceptance to these parts of you because they are asking for your attention and have been for a long time. Let that little girl or boy out of the locked room and give them a hug. They only ever knew how to scream, sulk, and kick to get your love.

1. Look for the self-critical voice saying some version of: *Do it better, don't do that, why do you always have to, or you should really . . .*

2. Smile internally, toward yourself.

3. Say, *You're already okay and getting better.*

4. Feel softness toward yourself because you are simply learning and discovering more and more, not fixing or repairing your mistakes.

### Travel Tip #3: Come Back into Your Body

One of the ways you have learned to protect yourself when you are encountering intense emotion is through *dissociation*, literally meaning leaving your body. Your body is the instrument of emotional transmission, and fragmenting off your awareness does not ultimately serve your feeling of wholeness. When you feel overwhelmed or know you are not present to what is happening before you because it feels like alarms are blaring inside, put your hands onto some area of your body. Touch your face, put a hand on your chest, run your fingers down the front of your body and say, *open, open, open* to consciously relax and release tension you may be accumulating in that area.

## THE WAY HOME

Hands down, the mantra of my practice, my online program, and my own personal journey is this: *I finally feel like myself.* Entirely changed perhaps, but closer to the essence of my being.

Over and over and over again, I hear this phrase: *I am becoming more and more myself. I am being liberated into my own truth and being-ness.* You look back on the path you have traveled, and you say, yes, it needed to be exactly this way. Nothing was bad. Nothing was wrong. Hard, maybe. Painful, sure. But I am not broken. I am not diseased. And nothing is a foregone conclusion or an absolute certainty.

Only you can know you are on the path of self-realization—to get real, get well, and get free. You will know when you're on it because you will feel the terrible pain and the glorious beauty of this life all at once, and you will feel—finally *feel*—yourself.

---

### Resetter: Beatrice

Personally, embarking on the Vital Mind Reset program has been nothing short of a beautiful surprise of discovery, mind, body, and spirit. From my relationships with my husband, family, friends, my approach toward infertility, my self-worth and acceptance, and a celebration of being curious and happy in my own skin, I am in awe of my life.

This feels like the portal for a new way of life. Looking back, I was living in a constant state of anxiety and fear, feeling unworthy, codependent, and gripped in a cycle of grief and unsettling insecurity. It was exhausting. Everything is different now, the veil of a cloudy, dark fog has lifted, and I know this is just the beginning.

---

C8∞

## What's Next . . .

For a deeper dive into the radical new perspective on mental health I'm describing, in Chapter 4 we'll look at a pervasive and tenacious root of psychiatric symptom prevalence in our lives, a belief system based on fear.

Chapter 4

# FEAR IS THE SICKNESS

*Everything you've ever wanted is on the other side of fear.*

— GEORGE ADDAIR

When we can move beyond fear of our symptoms into curiosity, we find that all illness—*without exception*—is the body's wisdom playing out in its own highly designed and incredibly personal way. But this shift in mindset requires a deeper understanding of how we have outsourced our embodied power to doctors. In this chapter, we will explore how fear has come to dominate our mindset about health, wreaking havoc through the *nocebo effect,* and how embracing a new narrative about the meaning of your health journey can pave the path to true healing.

## HOW WE'VE STOPPED TRUSTING OUR BODIES

The good news is that you are in control of your health destiny. The bad news is . . . you are in control of your health destiny.

Your body responds intelligently to what you perceive, believe, and intend more than to what is "really" happening, so if you are fearful, conditioned into a victim mindset, and expectant of continued patterns of negativity, you are more likely to have continued negative outcomes. Without fear, your body can do what it does naturally: recalibrate and become whole/healthy again. In this way, fear is the sickness, and your symptoms—their duration and severity—are the expression of your fear.

We have been led to believe that we can't trust and don't understand our bodies, and that we need an expert to help us manage them. We look for our *diagnoses*. The labels we get in a doctor's office—depression, generalized anxiety, bipolar disorder, chronic fatigue—are more than words. These are modern-day hexes with the power to bring about negative outcomes.

Such labels as depression, anxiety, and cancer are further empowered because our culture supports a belief that gives *meaning* to your perception of these observed signs and symptoms: namely, that they are bad, damning and dooming you beyond your ability to do anything about them.

We create that meaning as a collective, and then we pass it on and around. It seeps through our culture as a "meme," an idea spreading pervasively from one mind to another through writing, speech, gestures, secular rituals, or other imitable phenomena. These memes are like energetic swarms that can suck you up into them if you don't know how to orient around your own truth. This explains how we decide, together, *what it is* we will trust or be afraid of.

The list of fears we agree to is curated and maintained by the media, supported by the direct-to-consumer ads of media sponsors (think pharmaceutical companies' dramatic portrayals of suffering alleviated by their drugs), all to keep us continuously learning and relearning when—and around what—to activate our fear response. These messages come to us courtesy of the pharmaceutical industry, sponsoring upward of 70 percent of mainstream media. This includes so-called astroturfing campaigns (fake grassroots commentaries), smearing alternative and holistic platforms on social media and promoting these messages on seemingly independent journalistic outlets.

When we marinate in a sea of negative emotions, such as worry, regret, disappointment, grief—all stemming from the fear that we are living in a ticking time bomb of a body—we have no power to heal naturally and we can do nothing. The message is clear: *you are a victim.*

## NOCEBO POWER

Enter the *nocebo effect*, a name for this power of negative beliefs to inflict bodily harm. Understanding the nocebo effect, you will clearly see how belief and expectations are the greatest drivers of suffering.

As I explained in Chapter 3, the placebo effect shows how our belief that we are being treated by a legitimate intervention can actually improve our subjective experience, even the outcome. *Nocebo* is the opposite, translated loosely to "being harmed by expectations." But with nocebo, there is typically no sugar pill involved—just the power of the story you are telling yourself.

In the literature, such beliefs are referred to as *expectancy*. Perhaps the best illustration of the placebo effect in treating mental and mood disorders such as depression is a study done at Columbia University.[1] Patients who felt they were better on Prozac were told that they would be "randomized" to either continue the exact dose that had helped them or get a sugar pill. It turns out that both groups became depressed.

Yes, Mary, who took her same 40 mg on Tuesday and then again on Wednesday when the trial began, became depressed days later simply because of the possibility that she *could have* gotten the sugar pill placebo. The loss of benefit with the introduction of the *possibility* of being randomized to placebo is the *undoing* of the placebo effect, or the nocebo effect.

Here's another example of just how powerful expectation and the nocebo effect are: A groundbreaking study reported in the *New England Journal of Medicine* reveals that there is increased risk of death from heart-related causes during the week following a cancer diagnosis—regardless of whether the diagnosis was accurate.[2] After analyzing over 500,000 people aged 30 and older who were diagnosed with cancer over a 15-year period, researchers found the risk of suicide was up to 16 times higher and the risk of heart-related death 26.9 times higher one week following diagnosis versus those who were cancer free. The power of expectation is that strong.

It's possible that a doctor's negative attitude and beliefs surrounding a diagnosis can contribute to this outcome by infecting the patient with helplessness and hopelessness, two psychospiritual states at the very root of disease. My partner, Sayer Ji, on the health empowerment database and resource greenmedinfo.com, references a more ancient example of this as the practice known as "bone-pointing." This ritual involved a shaman pointing a bone at a person whose death was said to be imminent and from supernatural causes, resulting in the person actually dying from emotionally induced trauma. Our modern-day shamans are likewise hexing their patients when they hand them what's perceived as a death sentence with a cancer diagnosis, and sometimes even end up killing them before the cancer ever would have.

The translation of emotions to physiology is becoming less and less "woo woo" and more and more scientifically validated. A landmark study of women with breast cancer provides even more evidence by demonstrating the mechanism for the power of emotions to affect outcomes.[3] Researchers measured markers of inflammation called *cytokines* and correlated them with levels of emotional acceptance. Previous studies have found that cytokines are elevated in cancer patients and can contribute to symptoms of fatigue, chronic pain, and nausea that not only diminish a person's quality of life, but also sap physical resources needed to heal.[4] Unfortunately, the very experience of being diagnosed with cancer creates a surge of pro-inflammatory cytokines, a form of medical hexing.[5]

Emotional acceptance was defined as the process by which a person allows emotions, both positive and negative, to emerge and dissipate without attempts to control, change, or reject these emotions. Measuring the women's cytokines against their levels of self-acceptance, this breast cancer study found that this emotional state yielded lower levels of inflammatory cytokines.

Of note, it seems that males' responses depend more strongly on information given about placebo (i.e., intellectually driven responses), whereas women are more sensitive to conditioned responses (i.e., felt) in the context of nocebo. That is, female study subjects who merely witnessed another female reporting side effects from a medication were twice as likely to experience these side effects from a sugar pill/sham medication. This is referred to as "social modeling."

So if even our culturally conditioned beliefs about harm and vulnerability can influence our physiology, how should we understand this bodily response? Is your body really being tricked, or is it responding intelligently to what you perceive as a conflict, distress, or danger? I would say yes to the body's intelligence and go even further to say it is possible that an early, imprinted experience of fear—unprocessed and unacknowledged—is actually what seeds the symptoms that are then ultimately diagnosed as a "disease" or dis-*ease*. Yes, fear is the disease, and your symptoms are the messenger.

## UNEXPRESSED ANGER AS A DRIVER OF ILLNESS

*When the Body Says No* is Dr. Gabor Maté's opus on the ways in which stress drives illnesses such as autoimmunity and cancer. Inspired by the science supporting a cancer personality type, Maté makes the argument that people pleasers and those who otherwise suppress their own emotional needs in service of others are at particular risk for developing immune-related illnesses.

Turns out there is a particular kind of chronic stress related to this self-denial. These people are emotionally controlled by others. They are relegated to a subordinate position. Disempowered and helpless, targets for what my dear friend and women's health pioneer Dr. Christiane Northrup would call *energy vampires*.[6]

It appears that one of the true risk factors for some forms of cancer and autoimmunity is an experience of childhood trauma, acute or chronic, wherein survival is linked to conforming to expectations that are ultimately self-violating. In fact, Maté says that every single one of his patients has struggled with emotional repression as a coping style and that not one of them could answer *yes* to the following question: *"When, as a child, you felt sad, upset, or angry, was there anyone you could talk to—even when he or she was the one who had triggered your negative emotions?"*

I would come to the same conclusion about the patients I've worked with.

Maté defines repression as "dissociating emotions from awareness and relegating them to the unconscious realm," which "disorganizes and confuses our physiological defenses so that in some people these defenses go awry, becoming the destroyers of health rather than its protectors."

Incredible longitudinal research has supported the ability to predict with 75 to 78 percent accuracy those that have clinical evidence of cancer or who have died from it based on measures of repressed anger and long-lasting hopelessness. Turns out that a brave face isn't helping anyone.

To complicate matters, Maté cites data suggesting that seeming stress-free breast cancer patients are *more* likely to be dead at follow-up. Positive thinking and emotions are not the same as genuine joy, he clarifies. They are a distraction technique from the fuller arena of emotional terrain. They defy the meaning and importance of a range of "negative" emotions that inform our authentic self: a self that seems to require essential expression for vital health.

Maté writes: "Negative thinking allows us to gaze unflinchingly on our own behalf at what does not work. We have seen in study after study that compulsive positive thinkers are more likely to develop disease and less likely to survive. Genuine positive thinking—or more deeply, positive being—empowers us to know that we have nothing to fear from truth."[7]

The poet John Keats coined the term "negative capability" in 1817, to mean "when Man is capable of being in uncertainties, mysteries, doubts, without any irritable reaching after facts and reason."[8] What he perceived, hundreds of years ago, is that true vision requires embracing the paradox and uncertainty of life.

## FEAR AND YOUR SHADOW

What determines whether or not something strikes fear into our hearts? I believe it is the lens we look through: our perceptions.

When we are triggered into reactivity—or the patterned responses that we learned from childhood— it means that one of our existential wires is tripped: either our belief that the world is unsafe, that no one will be there for us when the going gets rough, or commonly, that our bodies are shameful, broken entities. Shame is such a powerful driving force of allopathic intervention that it's almost like we are throngs of injured kids running to the doctor and hospital with our arms up, saying, *Just love me! Just make this bad body right!*

Because we are not typically conscious of the strong childhood emotions that are driving our adult behavior, we live in a state of repression and projection, imagining the badness to be coming from outside of us rather than from our rejected, abused, neglected, and suppressed parts. As Robert Augustus Masters, author of *Bringing Your Shadow Out of the Dark*, would say, we have little intimacy or comfort with our emotional selves.

According to Masters, our "shadow" is our internal storehouse for the aspects of us that we've disowned or rejected, or are otherwise keeping in the dark. Everyone has a shadow, but not everyone knows their shadow. And the degree to which we don't know our shadow is the degree to which it influences, controls, and runs us.

In Chapter 8, "The Lens of Your Perception," I will show you how to work with your shadow, but for now, be aware of these signs of an unexamined shadow that can lead you to states of fear, stress, and illness:

- Knee-jerk and defensive reactions
- Feeling numb or frozen when called to respond
- Stuck in old relationship patterns
- Saying you're okay when you're not
- Hiding behind "positive" response to something that honestly bothers you
- Being overly critical of yourself
- Being unable to apologize for something clearly you did wrong

## A FEARLESS APPROACH

What might it be like to live an emergency-free life in which you have a fearless approach to symptoms and even crises? Specifically, to face an experience of depression, anxiety, insomnia, and even the most terrifying diagnoses such as cancer and infection with trust, courage, and curiosity?

In my practice and online program, individuals labeled with chronic illness from bipolar disorder to lupus to Crohn's disease to OCD heal their bodies, free their minds, and leave their labels and meds behind, for good. I believe that these outcomes are largely attributable to the container of fearlessness and the curiosity that is therefore fostered. I treat my patients like the capable adults I know they can be if their childself is not demanding they be coddled as hapless victims. In this container, the words "worry" and "concern" are eliminated from our shared vocabulary, and every aspect of the experience of symptoms becomes a meaningful message to interpret in the context of the patient's lifescape. Without fear, we are able to receive any and all of what comes, without resistance and with more open arms, allowing for dramatic reversals and expansions to unfold.

It is my belief—and the science of PNI backs this up—that our emotions tell our bodies when and how to manifest symptoms. Once symptoms are expressed, we are invited to respond to the symptoms themselves. Do we freak out and run to the ER? Or do we embrace the symptoms and ask questions of ourselves to work through the symptoms with interest and resolve?

Here's what one of my participants in my online program had to say about negative emotions and the potential for not running from them:

---

### Resetter: Beth

On Monday, I was exhausted from a day at work and then looking after my kids. I took myself to a quiet place to rest and be still and soon felt something uplifting in the feeling of being exhausted. It was quite extraordinary! It's the second time this week that I felt negative emotions and then they evolved into something very different.

Again, today we have had to face up to some bad financial circumstances, and I was feeling great fear about it. But when I just let it be, that feeling morphed into a very blissful state full of gratitude and peace. I was almost crying tears of joy. Every part of me was feeling, but in a good way. I feel I'm a step nearer to not being so scared of different emotional states.

---

In my practice/program, the most important criterion for clinical success is a shared belief system that supports the power of the body to heal when properly supported. This support comes in the form of a high level of self-care commitment but also a mindset that is aligned with the body's full potential and acceptance around what *is*. It is founded on trust and results in powerful fearlessness.

In many ways, fears that arise around health can be seen as tests of belief. It's easy to see a given circumstance as an exception, an extreme, or a one-time concession, but each and every health experience we are delivered is a dance with our own belief system and a reflection of the trust we have cultivated in our own bodies.

When you truly believe in your body's capacity and wisdom, with all of your being, then you will pass these tests with flying colors. When you are in the process of transforming, however, there may be a threshold of fear that leads you to violate your own stated philosophies or personal desires for your own health and well-being. One of the most critical tenets of growth is integration: bringing what you say, believe, and do into alignment. This involves identification of the ways in which we claim one thing and do another; for example, claiming to believe in the sacredness and emergent design of life but seeking to commandeer and manage the body with pharmaceuticals when sufficiently afraid.

Illnesses and community-cultivated fears (Zika! Swine flu! Ebola!) may reveal to us our blind spots and unintegrated zones. But in order to live life in the ever-coveted flow, we need to push ourselves beyond the comfort zones of our mind, shedding layers of story and ego in order to become all that much more ourselves.

This is why I hold space for med-free living. My friends, family, and patients know that I walk the walk. No meds, no how. That includes everything from pain killers to antibiotics to birth control to chemotherapy. I've seen too many patients who have been injured by pharmaceuticals or lost years of their lives to the arrested developmental space that medication left them to stagnate in.

The next time you reach for pharmaceutical intervention, consider these medications for what they truly are: corporate opportunity to profit from your disempowerment and elective membership in a church that views the body as broken, fragile, and objectively material.

**Antibiotics.** By far the most alluring of all the poisoned apples, antibiotics ride a mindset of fear while fostering the illusion of the quick fix. *What if my ear infection invades my brain? What if this pneumonia kills me? Or my UTI attacks my kidneys?* Talk to anyone who has suffered from *fluoroquinolone toxicity,* an adverse reaction to the antibiotic ciprofloxacin that causes nervous system and musculoskeletal damage and manifests as multi-symptom, often chronic, illness and you will understand how a simple round of antibiotics can change your life forever.[9]

We need to develop a deeper respect for what it is to support the body through a process of recalibration through infection. Any traditional pediatrician like my friend Dr. Larry Palevsky will tell you that we grow from our infectious illnesses and that there is probably more to the story than that bad bugs are bad. In fact, sneezing, vomiting, diarrhea, and sweating are all inbuilt mechanisms to mobilize cellular toxicants. Consider that getting sick could represent the efforts of a wise body to recalibrate and recruit your attention and support, not your fear and interference.

The reality is that patterns of symptoms that we call infections have a natural course with an inbuilt capacity for robust recovery, so we may be giving undue credit to antibiotics. This appears to be possible based on the published literature. For instance, a study on rhinosinusitis concluded, "The risks of potential side effects need to be weighed against the potential benefit that antibiotics give to the patient. This is especially pertinent as usage of the placebo has shown to be almost as efficacious as using the antibiotic therapy, and also much safer."[10]

A 2017 review references the increased risk of subsequent infection, including with antibiotic-resistant strains, in those who took antibiotics during travel, with unpredictable recovery rates that seem to get dismally worse with repeated antibiotic exposure: "Even short antibiotic exposures disrupt the gut microbiome up to a year or more, and repeated exposures appear to attenuate recovery from ever occurring."[11]

Similarly, up to a one-third reduction in biome diversity can persist for longer than six months, even after one short course of the popularly dispensed antibiotic Cipro.[12] This decrease in diversity can itself be a precursor to new illness. For instance, inflammatory bowel disease (IBD) is one of several chronic illnesses associated with low levels of beneficial bacteria.[13] Dysbiosis (imbalanced gut bacteria) is also a precursor to autoimmunity,[14] obesity, and weight gain.[15]

From slowed fracture healing[16] to acute liver injury,[17] antibiotics have effects at the cellular level beyond simply inducing dysbiosis. These include changes in up to 87 percent of gut metabolites functional in the gut, injury and destruction of mitochondria (the energy centers of the cell), and damage to gut tissue.[18]

**Birth control.** Living with unbalanced hormones is no way to live. But you need to get to the root of your hormonal imbalance—sugar addiction, thyroid sluggishness, constipation, or an overwhelmed liver. I took birth control pills for 12 years straight, believing they were Western medicine's gift to women. Turns out that this gift is something of a Trojan horse, as birth control strips us of essential nutrients, drives inflammation, and interferes with sex and thyroid hormones, hijacking the very systems that are responsible for our life force. You cannot take the hormones out of the woman without taking the *woman* out of the woman.

**Vaccines.** In no way personalized to the needs of *your* body— read: gender, age, weight, immunologic history, stress level, exposures, family history—vaccines are the sacred cow of an industry that leaves no room for informed consent or individualized approaches to wellness. You'll see in Chapter 5 that vaccines can be potential drivers of psychiatric struggles like depression. But know that the philosophical underpinnings of the vaccination program are predicated on an antiquated perspective: warring against and attempting to eradicate bad germs. With the advent of our understanding of the microbiome, psychoneuroimmunology, and epigenetics, science has left that childlike notion in the dust, and so should we.

**Tylenol and Advil.** Seemingly benign, over-the-counter pain killers take the edge off. Why suffer if you don't have to? Unfortunately, interfering with our fevers, aches, and pains comes with a cost. Tylenol is a liver toxicant of epic proportions, and Advil is a gut bomb whose true toxicity is just being revealed.

---

*Fear is an infectious disease. You can catch fear but you can't catch faith. That has to come from within.*

— NICHOLAS GONZALEZ, M.D.

---

My mentor, the late, great Dr. Nicholas Gonzalez, was a specific influence in my life who reinforced this fearless approach to illness. He helped blast away any residual carve-outs, any circumstances in which I might say, *Well, that* does *require conventional medicine.* As I studied his natural healing protocol, which enabled decades-long outcomes for terminal cancer patients, I knew that there was indeed nothing to be afraid of. Ever. And when patients who had otherwise been hexed by the medical establishment met with him, they too shed their fear in favor of faith in the body's capacity to self-regulate and heal, even if part of the healing looked like sickness. And they did heal, by the hundreds.

While Nick had a protocol based on personalized nutrition, detox, and supplementation (one that has greatly informed my own), it is possible that this protocol only fortified the body's self-healing response, and is not actually what healed the patient. Proponents of Dr. Ryke Geerd Hamer's German New Medicine (GNM) would support that possibility.[19] They argue that disease is actually *adaptive* and evidence of a healing process already underway. Dr. Hamer believed that psychic conflict, particularly shocking conflict that is perceived as distressing, gives rise to a corresponding physiologic process that includes changes in cellular proliferation of organs. This process spontaneously resolves (with the help of the inner microbiome) when the conflict is addressed such that the symptoms are not the beginning, but the resolution phase of the problem.

For example, according to German New Medicine, the symptoms of a urinary tract infection can represent the resolution of a "territorial conflict" where one felt either literally or emotionally encroached upon, violated, or unsure of where one's personal space begins and ends. The ancient response, on a brain level, is to ulcerate the lining of the urethra to allow for more urinary flow to "mark territory" with bacteria helping resolve tissue replenishment and healing in the symptom-active phase.

The most compelling aspect of German New Medicine is that it recontextualizes cancer and infection as nothing to be afraid of; rather, what we think of as illness is simply the body's secondary process of resolving the psychic injury of the cancer diagnosis itself. Even conventional medicine agrees that certain early-stage cancers, like DCIS (ductal carcinoma in situ) breast cancer, thyroid cancer, and prostate cancer, should be left alone, as the treatments do nothing to prolong life and instead are likely detrimental.[20] In fact, treatment with chemotherapy and radiation not only disrupts a complex process that requires supportive attention, but also it induces secondary harm, both psychically and physiologically.

The GNM perspective undermines widely held and entirely evidence-less assumptions around infectious contagion and cancer metastases, decimating the psychology of warfare against dangerous invasive microbes out to get us and big bad cancer that eats up our innocent victim body. When we interfere and war with the body, we keep the fight alive, and you can't win the battle against yourself.

## FEAR-BASED THEORIES OF INFECTION: A CHALLENGE

For me, preschool-level depictions of the immune system as a troop of soldiers fighting off the enemy germ invader have always inspired an internal eye roll, but it wasn't until my deep dive into the complexity of immunology that I came to understand that we know nothing of it. In fact, the vast majority of immunology is thoroughly and completely devoted to vaccinology.

Wait, vaccines must have beneficial effects if they produce antibodies, right? Antibodies have been deemed synonymous with disease protection, and we've even used a surrogate marker for claims that vaccines "work" in the laboratory setting, but is there actually any science for this? And do the antibodies produced upon vaccination actually bind to and inactivate disease-causing agents? What if antibodies are simply response elements that support the body's reaction to the many toxic chemicals in vaccines, ranging from detergents like polysorbate 80 to formaldehyde?

And what about contagion? It has never actually been proven that germs travel from one person to another and infect them. Germs as pathogens is a complex question that science has contributed rich literature to in the past two decades. But with the dawn of the microbiome—our inner ecology that reveals not only our harmonious relationship to but our dependency on the very microbes we have demonized—everything about orthodox medicine *should* have changed. Including the discovery of so-called viruses embedded in our own genomic material, calling into question whether or not viruses actually exist in the way we have assumed.

Has a discrete virus, deemed unable to exist independently, ever been visualized under electron microscopy, or are we still inferring? Research into our inner ecology now speculates that up to 8 percent of what we call human DNA may have been viral in origin; this is called the *virome*. Viral, meaning nucleic acids in a protein coat that require cells to replicate, essentially nonliving agents of genetic information transfer. As we understand more about how genetic information is passed between living entities, we may come to question the vectors we empowered with causal roles.

Transmission of effects can take many forms that we can understand when we step out of the box of conventional medicine. Does a yawn spread like germs supposedly do? What about women's menstrual cycles syncing up when they live together? Or the spread of fear-induced illness, which is strikingly demonstrated in a study in which women who were convinced that they were inhaling "contaminated air" got sick when they saw others getting sick from it—despite the fact that there was nothing wrong with the air.[21] Then there are people who only get symptoms of a cold when they believe themselves to be unwell at baseline. All of these situations bring the simplistic theory of germs spreading by physical pathogens alone into question.

I have come to believe that symptoms of infection are evidence that the body knows how to, and needs to, *eliminate*. Vomiting, diarrhea, sweating, coughing, sneezing, and runny noses all have exudative elimination in common. This likely also explains why so many of my patients and online participants develop cold after pneumonia after cold after bronchitis during and after their taper process: their immune systems are finally able to begin to mobilize stored toxicants.

As we sit in even more curious territory, what other assumptions have we made that have been disproven or remain unproven to date? Science can be a beautiful tool for discovery, but only if it is allowed to dispassionately acknowledge when a more complete picture is emerging. Another wise friend, Charles Eisenstein, wrote in his epic truth tome, *Ascent of Humanity*: "When we see germs as predators who seek to steal 'resources' from us for their own biological interest (survival and reproduction), then a rational response is to deny them those resources, to hide from the predators or fight them off—the fight-or-flight response. . . . If I believe, on the contrary, that there is some reason specific to my own body why the flu has infected me and not you, then the program of control doesn't make sense anymore."[22]

Sometimes all it takes is a friendly reminder that when you are aligned with your body—and truly make a truce with it—you can access limitless reservoirs of healing energy. This is the reclamation I am interested in, for all of us. Once we understand that our symptoms and illnesses have meaning, that they are sending us a message, and we trust our body's capacity to move through them when supported, we become unstoppable vessels of revolution in today's bio-control society.

## WHAT DOES FEARLESS HEALING LOOK LIKE?

If fear is the sickness, what is the cure? It's possible that it is as simple as a shift in mindset and a reframing of the felt experience of the body, in the journey and in the exquisite design of it all through our beliefs, our lived experience, and our outcomes. Here, we engage a new story, where no one is a victim of bad genes, bad luck, and an unwanted lifelong relationship with the pharmaceutical industry.

You have a choice to bring curiosity to this challenge, to support your body through it rather than interfere with it, and to uplift a sense of your truest self, which lies underneath the experience of physical healing. In this way, you put a soundtrack to your life that says, *Isn't this interesting* and *There's nothing to worry about,* and *You've got this* instead of one that says *But what if I don't,* and *Oh my God, I couldn't live with myself if . . .* and *What would everyone think if . . .* and *Why is this happening to me? It's so unfair.*

It's happening to you because it is a part of you. The experience of illness is so deeply meaningful and purposeful that it is, quite literally, showing you yourself. Don't fear it; embrace it.

My ultimate goal is to orient you around your story that speaks your truth. To give you access to new beliefs that are not fearful but trusting. If, for instance, you believe that challenges—and even adversity—happen for a reason, that the body has an innate wisdom, and that the cosmos operates under the principles of an elegant design, you will bend and flow with what comes. You bring curiosity to bear and live a life grounded in trust, allowing you to be emergency free.

To get there, you have to stop fighting the war. You have to relinquish your role as a victim dependent on a system that holds all the answers that you yourself don't have within. When we look, we see wartime narratives embedded throughout our consciousness: "fighting" depression, cancer, and germs. But that war is never won, just perpetuated by constant resistance born of fear and the call to impose more and more control where measures of control have already failed and made the seeming problem worse. The end of war is not to keep on fighting. It is to give up fighting.

Worry serves nothing. In fact, it perpetuates that stress response that may be driving the entire health struggle. Ask what needs to be exposed, honored, balanced. Then find the approach, the medicine, or the healing that speaks to what you learn about your deepest needs for this lifetime. Accept the invitation to get real with yourself, get well, and get free so you can start over and finally experience the wonder of being fully expressed and who you truly are.

---

### Resetter: Robin

I had a funny experience today that shows how the body knows what to do once you give it time to reset. I'm on day two of a bad cold and thinking of what to eat. I was craving yogurt (nondairy, no sugar) and thought I would make a mushroom omelet, something I don't think I've ever made. Then I read that yogurt, mushrooms, eggs, and yams are some of the best ways to shorten a cold's length. So cool my body was craving all that!

---

## Travel Tip: When in Fear, Meditate

Try this meditation when you're experiencing fear:

### Meditation for a Calm Heart

- **Posture:** Sit cross-legged with a light neck lock (stretch the back of the neck upward to bring the chin slightly down and back). Place the left hand on the center of the chest at the heart center. The palm is flat against the chest, and the fingers are parallel to the ground, pointing to the right.

  Make gyan mudra with the right hand (touch the tip of the index finger with the tip of the thumb). Raise the right hand up to the right side as if giving a pledge. The palm faces forward, and the three fingers not in gyan mudra point up.

The elbow is relaxed near the side with the forearm perpendicular to the ground.

- **Eyes:** Either close the eyes or look straight ahead with the eyes one-tenth open.
- **Breath:** Inhale slowly and deeply through both nostrils. Then suspend the breath in and raise the chest. Retain it for as long as possible. Then exhale smoothly, gradually, and completely. When the breath is totally out, lock the breath out for as long as possible.

  Concentrate on the flow of the breath. Regulate each bit of the breath consciously.

- **To end:** Inhale and exhale strongly three times. Relax.[23]

CB BO

## What's Next . . .

In Part II, you will get a chance to shift from fear to fearlessness through a felt experience of the innate power and wisdom of your body. From my perspective, the best place to start is with meditation, detox, and high-integrity nutrition, the elements of my one-month healing protocol that you will learn about in Part II.

But before you begin and take on a one-month challenge, you'll want to read in Chapter 5 about how to know if your symptoms are caused by or related to what I call the "psychiatric pretenders," five physical conditions that mimic the symptoms of mental disorders. Only then can you manage your symptoms more holistically, treating all possible causes.

# GET
# WELL

Chapter 5

# FROM MESS TO MEANING: FIVE PSYCHIATRIC "PRETENDERS"

*Your body's ability to heal is greater than anyone has permitted you to believe.*

— UNKNOWN SOURCE

Having read this far, you now know that so-called mental illness is far from simply a brain chemical imbalance. Behind the label of a diagnosis is the real root cause toward which your body is calling your attention, and when you get curious and look into that cause—turning toward your body instead of fighting it—you can begin your healing journey. In my experience, the vast majority of symptoms, from brain fog to fatigue to poor concentration; flat or erratic mood to panic attacks, obsessive behavior, and anxiety, can be addressed by starting with a focus on healing the body. You can better address what's left in the emotional and psychospiritual realms after a strong physical foundation is established.

Let's begin by taking a look at some of mental illness's common disguises: the physical imbalances that can masquerade as mental illnesses. We will explore in depth how your body is communicating with you through your physical symptoms—tapping you on the shoulder and saying, *Hey, look in here!* We'll cover the many ways in which "mental illness" is actually a label put on a bodily request to pay attention and change the way you are living, day to day.

## THE GREAT PRETENDERS

The good news is that textbook psychiatric disorders can actually represent some very ordinary physical imbalances that are routinely undiagnosed. They are what I call the *psychiatric pretenders*, five physiologic conditions that can leave you with symptoms that are indistinguishable from depression and other so-called mental disorders.

For example, an unbalanced thyroid—*not* unbalanced brain chemicals—is among the most common "pretenders" in women today. In fact, *hypothyroidism* (an overwhelmed and thus underperforming thyroid) is one of the most underdiagnosed conditions in America.

Four other pretenders round out the picture of why you shouldn't accept a diagnosis of a mood or mental disorder without investigating the source of your symptoms. These are 1) gluten (and dairy) sensitivity, 2) blood sugar instability, 3) vitamin $B_{12}$ deficiency, and 4) medication effects. Because of this complexity, the psychiatric diagnosis handed to you could have you taking Zoloft for an endocrine condition or Lamictal for a $B_{12}$ deficiency—not intelligent medicine.

## PRETENDER #1: THYROID DYSFUNCTION

The vast majority of symptoms that occur with a thyroid disorder could easily come under a "depression" diagnosis. Most of us never think about our thyroid, but this butterfly-shaped gland located at the base of the neck has important functions, including playing a key role in metabolism, digestion, elimination, appetite, energy, temperature, sleep, and mood. Hypothyroidism occurs when the thyroid gland is underactive because of nutrient deficiency or inflammation and doesn't produce enough thyroid hormone.

Specifically, the thyroid is responsible for producing hormones called T0, T1, T2, T3, and T4. The two most active thyroid hormones are T3 and T4. Most of the T4, the storage form of thyroid hormone, is converted into its active form, T3, in tissues around the body including the brain. This conversion to active thyroid hormone is dependent on specialized enzymes, optimal cortisol (your stress hormone), and certain nutrients such as iron, iodine, zinc, magnesium, selenium, B vitamins, vitamin C, and vitamin D.

In our fast-paced, nutrient-depleted world filled with toxic substances, this one hormonal conversion step alone can be easily impaired. And while you may not feel the attack in your thyroid per se, you'll definitely feel it in your mood, energy, and cognition. When the thyroid is responding to stressors, you can experience an array of depression-like symptoms, including fatigue, constipation, hair loss, low mood, foggy thinking, feeling cold all the time, low metabolism, weight gain, dry skin, muscle aches, and an intolerance for exercise. You're wearing socks to bed, pooping only once a week, and penciling in your eyebrows because the hair has gone missing.

And then there's the special consideration of postpartum thyroiditis, a condition that 10 percent of women develop after delivery. It's a condition that I was diagnosed with nine months after the birth of my first child, and one that invited me to reexamine my lifestyle, and then later my entire life. This is whole-person medicine.

Interestingly, a recent study demonstrated that treatment with synthetic prescription hormone (levothyroxine or Synthroid) did not actually resolve associated depression, arguing for root cause resolution and whole body treatment over symptom management.[1]

---

### Resetter: Sam

My endocrinologist said my thyroid condition (Graves' disease) looks to be in remission. I completed the Reset program, and now he's lowered my medication a second time. I love that my labs are a testament that I am getting better—a big surprise to my doctor, who told me in our first appointment that Graves' was strictly an autoimmune disease and diet would make no difference. He also told me my thyroid played no part in my past mental illness . . . Ha, ha, *yeah right!*

---

## NATASCHA'S STORY: REVERSAL OF GRAVES' DISEASE

Like Hashimoto's, Graves' disease is an autoimmune condition in which the immune system responds to perceived danger by hyperstimulating the thyroid gland.

Natascha came to me for relief from the following symptoms: night sweats, hair loss, tearfulness, forgetfulness, palpitations, weight loss, agitation, low libido, and vaginal dryness. She also reported one to two months of very low mood and hopelessness. My prescription? An anti-inflammatory/ancestral diet, advice to minimize toxicant/environmental exposures, and encouragement to eat natural fats for brain support.

Having confronted surgical removal of this precious gland, Natascha had this to say after completing her program: "I'm feeling a lot better than I did, even many years before my diagnosis with Graves' disease. I'm so grateful that I could save my thyroid and regain my health. To find that my body had my back all along was the most empowering and amazing feeling in the world. Just by giving it a little more of what it needed, it bounced back beautifully."

The dramatic healing of Natascha's Graves' disease with dietary modification, meditation, and detox will soon be reported as a precedent-setting case study in a peer-reviewed journal.

Healing the gut means eliminating specific food antigens, but almost always gluten. My protocol with a strong gluten-free emphasis in Chapter 6 can help return thyroid function to normal and quiet the immune system. This can be done with or without lab test verification, since the Reset is a comprehensive starting point for all of these imbalances.

Let's turn now to the second "pretender" that is diagnosed as a psychiatric disorder when it is not—gluten sensitivity.

## PRETENDER #2: GLUTEN AND CASEIN SENSITIVITY

It's estimated that up to 80 percent of the population has some sort of intestinal permeability and gut microbe deficiency, which can make digesting the proteins found in wheat especially problematic.

With a growing body of research linking gluten to various inflammatory disorders, "non-celiac gluten sensitivity" is on the rise.

Through the gut-brain axis, symptoms can include brain fog, fatigue, depression, migraines, and a host of other psychiatric symptoms. This is in addition to skin rashes, bone or joint pain, bloating, and/or weight loss. Over time this can cause antibodies to be formed against brain and other tissues.

Gluten, from the Latin word for "glue," is a composite of proteins consisting of *gliadin* and *glutenin*, both found in wheat. When I suggest eliminating gluten to patients, they sometimes tell me that they have already been tested and "don't have celiac." The limitations of conventional testing are very real, as most physicians who do a "celiac panel" are only testing for a small portion of the potential immune responses to this food. In one preliminary study, inflammatory response was noted in healthy volunteers, suggesting that gluten may cause reactions in *everyone*.[2]

If you're skeptical about the benefit of going gluten free, but open to it, a case reported in the *New England Journal of Medicine* suggests that, yes, gluten is an issue and not a wellness fad.[3] It goes so far as to say that dietary elimination of gluten may very well be the key to resolving what would otherwise be a chronic and disabling psychiatric condition, offering the following case report.

**Case study.** A 37-year-old woman who was studying for an advanced degree and who was under a lot of stress began expressing the belief that people were talking about her. This belief progressed to paranoia when, a few months later, her home was burglarized, and she accused her parents of conspiring to rob her.

The woman was hospitalized at a state psychiatric facility where she was labeled with psychotic disorder. She was treated with the drugs risperidone and sertraline and then discharged after one month. She was ultimately diagnosed with Hashimoto's as well as celiac disease, which accounted for her multiple nutrient deficiencies, weight loss, and inability to absorb thyroid hormone medication.

After receiving the diagnosis of celiac disease, she thought her practitioners were being deceitful regarding the diagnosis and refused to adhere to a gluten-free diet. Psychotic symptoms and paranoia persisted, and she continued to "find clues" of conspiracy against her. She lost her job, became homeless, and attempted suicide; her family had to take out a restraining order against her. Eventually, she was rehospitalized at an inpatient psychiatric facility, where she was placed on a strict gluten-free diet.

After three months, her delusions resolved completely and were associated with remission of celiac. At the time of the case write-up, she had relapsed psychiatrically after an inadvertent exposure to gluten.

From this report showing the gluten-brain connection, it would seem that a trial of a strict gluten-free diet for anyone presenting with symptoms of psychiatric and neurologic illness would be a good idea. Especially in light of increasing acknowledgment of non-celiac gluten sensitivity, not just celiac disease, having a very real psychiatric manifestation including depression and psychosis.

Why and how would these foods cause the problems that they do? A fascinating study helps elucidate just how wheat/gluten grains can promote intestinal permeability or "leaky gut," allowing peptides through this precious barrier where they go on to stimulate the brain and immune system.[4] A concept referred to as "molecular mimicry" underlies the direct relationship between these peptides and immune response agents that end up attacking tissues that share amino acid sequences with the offending intruder (e.g., a bagel).

Furthermore, digested proteins from cow dairy and gluten, termed *exorphins*, interact with opiate receptors in the brain, which accounts for the potentially addictive quality of these foods and the associated withdrawal when they are taken off the menu. Sayer Ji of greenmedinfo.com details the history dating back to 1951 of gluten in psychiatric and specifically psychotic illness.[5] More recent data has demonstrated that patients with a diagnosis of schizophrenia are two to three times as likely to have immune reactivity to wheat.[6]

Essentially, going gluten free should mean eliminating processed food from your life, which is why I also recommend elimination of co-reactive foods like corn, soy, and in some cases legumes (including peanuts), and gluten-free grains like rice and millet. I also recommend elimination of dairy to include all milk-based foods and products including yogurt, cheese, and ice cream, due to the protein *casein*.

Casein is the name for a family of proteins found in mammalian milk. It is possible that our modern, post-industrial foods—gluten and processed dairy, as well as sugar and genetically modified soy and corn—are conspiring with nutrient deficiencies in an incendiary collaboration that gives rise to gut/brain pathology.

The molecular similarity between gluten and casein makes them coconspirators. However, dairy immune provocation appears to be more variable from person to person. In cow dairy, there are six types of protein: four casein, making up 80 percent, and two whey. Within the casein category, A1-beta casein is most commonly present in American cows (Holstein) and is thought to represent a mutated form of the protein, only 5,000 years old. *Casomorphin*, an opiate-stimulating compound, is released from A1-beta casein. A2-beta casein is found in the milk of sheep, goats, and Jersey cows.

Researchers have also identified elevated antibodies to alpha, kappa, and whole casein in new-onset and treated schizophrenic patients.[7] In patients with casein antibodies, there was a seven to eight times increase in the diagnosis of schizophrenia, and they have similarly demonstrated a three to five times increased risk of bipolar disorder in patients with casein antibodies (IgG).

Beyond direct brain stimulation and poor digestion with local inflammation, cow dairy may also be a source of folate antibodies, which can gum up receptors responsible for transporting this critical nutrient to the brain.

It is my firm conviction that diet—both what it may be deficient in and its potential toxicity—can cause what we label as mental illness. My strongest mandate as a psychiatrist is that of a gluten- and casein-free dietary trial. Only then can these pretenders be unmasked and not diagnosed as mental illness.

In Chapter 6, I'll show you how you can do that dietary trial, supported by my one-month Reset protocol, which is also available as an online program.

## PRETENDER #3: BLOOD SUGAR INSTABILITY

One of the most effective ways to heal a dysfunctional immune system and thyroid gland—and their effect on your mental health—is by eliminating processed sugar to get your blood sugar under control. You read that right: the secret to ending your mood, behavioral, and cognitive symptoms could very well be in stopping the highs and lows (the sugar roller coaster) that are taking place in your bloodstream and, by implication, your brain.

*Reactive hypoglycemia* is a blood sugar imbalance that occurs after eating. When a person consumes high amounts of sugar (either through obvious forms like soda, or non-obvious forms like pasta), blood sugar increases quickly. This fast increase then spikes insulin, and blood sugar crashes. This forces cortisol to compensate and try to move sugar out of storage and back into the bloodstream.

Over time, this process is responsible for carb and sugar cravings (since in the non-breatharians among us, the brain needs a steady supply of sugar to function), which can frequently result in feeling "hangry" after skipping a meal. This can also lead to anxiety, irritability, headaches, dizzy spells, and trouble sleeping. Balancing blood sugar chaos may also save you from a diagnosis of panic disorder, generalized anxiety, symptoms associated with ADHD diagnoses, and even bipolar disorder, and keep you from relying on medication that can inflict harm on your mind and body.

Here's a typical scenario. You wake up, have a glass of orange juice and a bagel (or a bowl of "healthy" cereal, or a Special K bar), and your pancreas is confronted with a wave of sugar that it does not react kindly to. It puts out a counterwave of insulin, charged with sweeping that sugar into cells for energy production. The resultant dip in blood sugar can alarm the body and the adrenal glands, making them work overtime. These glands are charged with producing cortisol (which ultimately promotes *insulin resistance* or the lack of cellular response to insulin) and fight-or-flight chemicals that can get your heart racing and ratchet up anxiety. The solution to this agitated slump is often a follow-up serving of refined carbohydrate and/or caffeine and sugar—midmorning cookie with coffee.

The more days of your life you engage in this pattern of sugar and refined carb consumption, the more your brain suffers, potentially even putting you at risk for Alzheimer's dementia down the line, according to my esteemed colleague Dr. David Perlmutter.[8,9]

The solution is to restore sugar balance by eliminating sugar and refined flours from the diet and incorporating more protein and natural fats, particularly for breakfast. It's also a good idea to eat every two and a half hours—sometimes for a period of months or even years—until this response has had a chance to correct itself.

## JESSICA'S STORY: PMS AND INSOMNIA, OR BLOOD SUGAR IMBALANCE?

Jessica, 23, came to me due to premenstrual syndrome (PMS) with acne and a pervasive sense of unease that qualified as textbook depression. She frequently woke up in the middle of the night to snack but wasn't hungry when she dragged herself out of bed in the morning. This little tidbit was enough to tell me that her blood sugar balance was a distant memory. She also mentioned nagging fogginess, low energy, a low libido, and racing heart—all details that further clued me in to her blood sugar mayhem.

Within just a few weeks of dietary change, she had lost eight pounds and was sleeping through the night for the first time in four years, and she had no menstrual complaints by her third cycle. The ongoing anxiety that had clouded her days had disappeared.

We aren't designed to eat the amounts and types of sugars we are consuming today, some of which are hidden in seemingly innocuous foods marketed as healthy (such as whole-grain, complex-carbohydrate cereals, low-fat yogurts, and diet sodas containing artificial sugars). The reaction that takes place in the body in response to this high intake of various forms of sugar can masquerade as a number of different symptoms consistent with depression and anxiety. And these feelings can last all throughout the day, week, or month, contributing to a general sense of unease and agitation that might land you in your doctor's office, with her handing you a prescription for an antidepressant.

Thankfully there's a simple resolution to this, which we'll explore in Chapter 6: eliminating those abusive sugars and refined flours, and consuming more high-quality natural fats, especially at breakfast.

## PRETENDER #4: B$_{12}$ DEFICIENCY

Vitamin B$_{12}$ plays a critical role throughout the body and is associated with improved energy levels, improved moods, and healthy nervous system function. A deficiency of this key nutrient is extremely common, however, especially for those with compromised gut health, small bowel inflammation, and/or autoimmune disease.

Vitamin B$_{12}$ is among the most important vitamins when it comes to depression and mental health. Here are some of the reasons that vitamin B$_{12}$ is so important: B$_{12}$ supports myelin, the sheath around nerve fibers that allows nerve impulses to conduct. So when this vitamin is deficient, it's suspected of driving symptoms such as an impaired gait, loss of sensation, signs of dementia and even multiple sclerosis. But what about B$_{12}$'s role in psychiatric symptoms such as depression, anxiety, fatigue, and even psychosis?

The role of Vitamin B$_{12}$ in neuropsychiatric syndromes can best be explained by two basic biological mechanisms:

**Methylation.** Methylation is the process of taking a single carbon and three hydrogens, known as a methyl group, and applying that group to countless critical functions in your body, such as thinking, repairing DNA, turning on and off genes, building and metabolizing neurotransmitters, producing energy and cell membranes, and getting rid of environmental toxins, to name a few. DNA methylation in particular is the process of marking genes for expression rather than silencing them.

**Homocysteine recycling.** Vitamin B$_{12}$ is a primary player in the recycling of a compound that can be inflammatory when it builds up: *homocysteine.* In other words, vitamin B$_{12}$ is necessary to keep homocysteine in check. High homocysteine levels are typically found in those who suffer from depression. High levels are also a marker for heart disease and stroke risk.

One of the most remarkable papers I have read in the psychiatric literature was about a 57-year-old woman who was treated for months with both antipsychotic and antidepressant medications and given two rounds of electroconvulsive treatment before anyone bothered to check her vitamin B$_{12}$ level.[10] Her symptoms, years in the making, including tearfulness, anxiety, movement abnormalities, constipation, lethargy, and eventually perceptual disturbances (hearing her name called) and the ultimate in severe psychiatric pathology: catatonia. Despite her inpatient treatment, she remained suicidal, depressed, and lethargic. Within two months of identifying her deficiency, and subsequent B$_{12}$ treatment, she reverted to her baseline of 14 years previous, and remained stable with no additional treatment. With some two-fifths of the population presenting with severe deficiency, we must ask how they became deficient in the first place.[11] One cause could be low stomach acid.

**Low stomach acid** sometimes occurs in the setting of low thyroid function, chronic stress, aging, and most salient to a recent study, acid-blocking medications (think Prilosec, Nexium, Prevacid, and Protonix) taken to avoid indigestion or acid reflux (gastroesophageal reflux disease, or GERD).[12] Stomach acid is critical for triggering digestive enzymes, along with an escort called *intrinsic factor* for vitamin B$_{12}$ absorption, and for managing local microbial populations. So if you become deficient in B$_{12}$ and digestive imbalance goes unattended, you will likely develop symptoms that could lead to a prescription for an antidepressant.

## PRETENDER #5: MEDICATION REACTIONS

This bears repeating: there's no free lunch with medications. We've all listened to the ticker tape of side effects—including blindness and death—reported by TV commercials for pharmaceuticals. But how many medications have been causally linked (with known mechanisms) to entirely reversible psychiatric diagnoses and symptoms? More than you've been told. It may very well be that symptoms of anxiety, depression, inattention, fatigue, insomnia, and worse are actually means of the body saying *no* to a given medication exposure.

I want to set the record straight on "non-psychiatric" drugs that can trigger symptoms of depression, especially in cases of multiple prescriptions, a troubling trend labeled *polypharmacy*. Then I'll report on two of the drugs you may never think to associate with mental health: birth control pills and statins. I'll include a few more problematic drugs that are all too common in people's medicine cabinets today—Tylenol and Advil (nonsteroidal anti-inflammatory drugs, or NSAIDs)—and end with a highly cautionary note about the depression link to antibiotics and vaccines.

## POLYPHARMACY AND DEPRESSION

A Mayo Clinic study found that 7 out of 10 Americans take at least one prescription drug,[13] and a 2017 *Consumer Reports* survey found that over 55 percent of Americans regularly take four prescriptions on average.[14] This means that more than half of us are existing daily under the influence of *polypharmacy*; that is, simultaneously using multiple medications, day after day.

Here's what makes all this very bad news: a common polypharmacy side effect is depression. A 2018 University of Chicago study was the first to demonstrate that simultaneous use of prescription medications is associated with a greater likelihood of experiencing depression.[15] In fact, researchers found that more than one-third of U.S. adults are taking at least one medication that can trigger depression.

And worse, they probably don't even know it. Many may be surprised to learn that the medications they're currently taking, despite having nothing to do with mood disturbance or any other condition associated with depression, can increase their risk of experiencing depression.

The three I'll examine here are birth control pills, statins, and common pain killers such as Tylenol and Advil.

---

**Resetter: Rico**

My last psychiatrist was actually disciplined for putting me on a toxic combination of medications. My intuition told me I was taking too much, but when I questioned him, he told me my reaction was due to my mental health declining, not his wrong prescribing.

I have gone from being fearful of all intense emotions to now being excited for my life and what's to come. It feels amazing to simply feel into my feelings after being numb for so long—I'm so grateful for every feeling that I have. I can finally say that I have come home to my true self, who I have complete love for.

---

**Birth control pills.** When patients come to me with complaints of low libido, low or flat mood, weight gain, hair loss, and cloudy thinking, one of my first questions is, Are you on the Pill? When they complain about premenstrual irritability, insomnia, tearfulness, bloating, and breast tenderness, requesting that I sanction a course of oral contraceptives combined with an antidepressant, I tell them there's a better way.

Since the 1960s, there has been controversy surrounding the potential mood effects of oral contraceptives, but more than 50 years of use has not settled this question. There are pilot studies that demonstrate women using the oral contraceptive pill are significantly more depressed than a matched group who do not—something I see firsthand, most notably in those who begin contraception (hormonal IUD, progestin only, or combined) postpartum.[16]

And we know that depression is the most common reason for discontinuation of use. The data suggests overall that there is a subset of women for whom oral contraceptives represent a major risk factor for depression and/or related mood disturbance. Who might these women be? From 13 prospective trials, it appears that these are younger women who have a personal or family history of having been psychiatrically diagnosed, particularly related to pregnancy/postpartum.[17]

We now have the largest epidemiologic study of its kind, published in *JAMA*, in which one million women ages 15 to 34 were followed for 13 years.[18] Here's what they found:

- Women who were prescribed the combined pill (progestin and estrogen) were 23 percent more likely to be treated with antidepressants.

- Progestin-only treated women (sometimes called the "mini pill") were 34 percent more likely.

- Teens were 80 percent more likely if prescribed the combined pill and twice as likely with the progestin-only pill.

While the mood risks of hormonal contraceptives are well known, little attention has been paid to the life-threatening potential side effect of suicide. A 17-year Danish study published in 2017 has revealed a startling association between hormonal contraception and the risk of suicide and suicide attempts in women from ages 15 to 33.[19] These previously mentally healthy women had no prior history of suicide attempts, psychiatric diagnoses, or antidepressant use.

One of the most startling revelations from the Copenhagen research was that the relative risk of suicide attempt doubled just one month after first use of hormonal contraceptives. What could so quickly turn a nonsuicidal person into a suicidal one?

The Copenhagen researchers suggest that one explanation for the increased risk in suicidal behaviors is that hormonal contraceptives likely have a direct influence on brain structures involved in stress regulation and the neurobiology of suicidal behaviors.[20]

Following are some more of the most important findings of the 2017 Copenhagen study about suicide risk:

- Adolescents are at greatest risk because adolescence is a period characterized by hormonal changes that could exacerbate the influence of any additional factor (such as hormonal contraceptives) that might cause mood disturbances.

- Former hormonal contraceptive use was associated with an increased risk of suicide attempt and suicide.

Interestingly, a Mayo Clinic study found that the rate of suicide in the general population was less than .05 percent for those with no previous history of mental illness, much lower than the statistical risk of suicide for women who use hormonal contraceptives.[21]

If you're taking birth control for your hormonal imbalance, then heal your body. Start with food and add detox and meditation in the ways I will show you in Chapter 6. When you balance your hormones naturally, you learn that a woman's experience is cyclical. Energies shift to particular rhythms, and you can watch yourself to know exactly when in your life you're supposed to be doing what. It's called getting in touch with yourself, and it's what true empowerment is all about.

---

### Resetter: Lynne

I first joined the online program in hopes of it getting rid of my brain fog. I thought it also might allow me to taper off my anti-anxiety med. I never in a million years imagined that I would taper off my mood stabilizer as well. And so much changed: my body, mind, feelings, and self-confidence all changed. My PMS went from days of raging anger and anxiety and frustration to my period showing up without a sign. My actual hormones changed because of me following this Reset program.

---

**Statins: cholesterol-lowering drugs.** Chances are you or someone you know takes a cholesterol-lowering drug such as Crestor, Lipitor, or Zocor, assuming it will help prevent a fatal heart attack. Recent guidelines have expanded the number of potential statin users, adding 13 million new people to the pool of candidates for statin treatment.[22]

But you may not know how statins can affect your brain. New research reveals that statins may lessen brain function and increase risk for diabetes, heart disease, and depression. The reason is simple: the body and brain both need cholesterol in order to thrive. Reams of scientific data show time and time again that extremely low cholesterol levels are linked to depression, memory loss, and even violence toward oneself and others.[23]

Furthermore, it has been known for almost 30 years that low levels are associated with habitually violent tendencies of homicidal offenders under the influence of alcohol.[24] Since then, many studies have either confirmed or explored the cholesterol-violence link, including violence toward both self and others.[25]

A review article called "Neuropsychiatric Adverse Events Associated with Statins" discusses the state of the literature around the intersection between mental health and cholesterol control and concludes that severe irritability, homicidal impulses, threats, road rage, depression and violence, paranoia, alienation, and antisocial behavior have all been reported in registries of those taking statin medications.[26] The signal for certain statins—simvastatin and atorvastatin—was stronger. These medications penetrate the brain, and brain cholesterol deficiency has been implicated in bipolar disorder, major depression, and schizophrenia.

**Fat-slamming and brain health.** Since the 1950s, we've been told that eating fat makes you fat and that avoiding traditional fats (butter, animal meats, and eggs) in lieu of industrialized, man-made fats (margarine) is highly recommended. As a result, we have suffered ever-escalating rates of chronic inflammatory diseases like diabetes and the very heart disease we were aiming to prevent. But if you are struggling with hormonal imbalance and mood symptoms, you might want to know that cholesterol is a vital nutrient for brain health, a fact that has gotten lost amid all the fat-slamming. It turns out that 25 percent of the total amount of cholesterol found in the human body is localized in the brain, 70 percent of it in the myelin sheath that coats and insulates the nerves. By extension, behavioral and cognitive adverse effects may be the manifestation of this fat-based interference.

In a powerful expert review, researchers Diamond and Ravnskov state: "A low serum cholesterol level has also been found to serve as a biological marker of major depression and suicidal behavior, whereas high cholesterol is protective." In their review, they decimate any plausible indication for cholesterol-lowering agents, giving full consideration to the above-mentioned side effects. They plainly state: "Overall, our goal in this review is to explain how the war on cholesterol has been fought by advocates that have used statistical deception to create the appearance that statins are wonder drugs, when the reality is that their trivial benefit is more than offset by their adverse effects."[27]

As my patients' lab results come in, I often note that those with mood symptoms invariably have a fasting cholesterol below 160. Their internists may be impressed and pleased with their low-fat diets, but I'm not.

The body also recruits cholesterol to produce *pregnenolone*, a molecule that's a precursor to sex hormones such as testosterone and estrogen, so without it our reproductive and endocrine systems go awry. Think libido, harmonious menstrual cycle, clear skin, balanced metabolism, and cognition. Additionally, vitamin D, a steroid-like wonder hormone, is produced from cholesterol precursors, and its deficiency appears to be correlated with maladies too numerous to mention (but, yes, including depression).

**Common pain killers: Tylenol and other NSAIDs.** Prescription meds are not the only culprits in the polypharmacy-depression link, according to the previously cited 2018 study.[28] A 2017 *Consumer Reports* survey found that 75 percent of people taking prescription medication also take at least one over-the-counter drug regularly, which further increases the risk of adverse drug effects.[29]

*Just take a Tylenol.* This might as well be the American mantra. It's the perspective that we have been indoctrinated to adopt—that our bodies are full of annoying symptoms that can be suppressed by drugs.

The main ingredient in Tylenol is *acetaminophen*, which has been used in the United States for more than 70 years. It's considered a benign over-the-counter medication, used reflexively for aches, pains, and fever, and is widely thought of as safe for pregnancy. About 23 percent of American adults (about 52 million people) use a medicine containing acetaminophen each week. It's the most common drug ingredient in the United States, found in more than 600 medicines, but this "harmless drug" is linked to over 110,000 injuries and deaths per year.[30]

How can Tylenol, which is doled out like candy, be bad for you? Amazingly, no one really knows how acetaminophen works,[31] but people do know that this drug gets to your brain. Tylenol in your brain is concerning because it depletes glutathione, an antioxidant that is especially necessary for brain health.[32] Our bodies depend on antioxidants to balance oxidative damage and inflammation.

Most people have heard that Tylenol can damage the liver (has anyone ever drunkenly warned you to take a Motrin, not a Tylenol, to prevent a hangover?). But since everything in your body is connected, it's not surprising that Tylenol can do damage beyond your liver. After swallowing 1,000 mg of Tylenol, people exhibited less empathy and blunted positive emotions.[33] For reference, 1,000 mg is two extra-strength Tylenol tablets, and the "safe" range is 3,000 mg per day. This means that popping two Tylenols can affect you physically and emotionally in ways that are just starting to be elucidated.

Hopefully you're convinced to think twice before taking a Tylenol, but what about other pain relievers like Motrin, Aleve, or Advil? These nonsteroidal anti-inflammatory drugs (NSAIDs) must be safe, since 30 million people take them every day! Not so fast . . .

Women who recognize the importance of hormonal balance should be wary. NSAIDs can mess with ovulation, especially progesterone levels, after only 10 days of use.[34]

Additionally, NSAIDs injure the small intestine; in one study, 71 percent of NSAID users showed small intestinal damage, compared to 10 percent of nonusers.[35] Damaged intestines can lead to intestinal permeability, or "leaky gut" or gut permeability, which is linked to depression, ADHD, and allergies, as was discussed in Chapter 1. NSAIDs can induce leaky gut and harm your microbiome, the inner ecology of organisms you rely on for wellness.[36]

## PSYCHIATRIC SIDE EFFECTS OF ANTIBIOTICS AND VACCINES

**Antibiotics.** We are just beginning to unravel the hows and whys of antibiotic effects on the brain. Invented and studied before our knowledge of the microbiome and the role of mitochondrial dysfunction in chronic disease, antibiotics have long been reported to have psychiatric side effects but have never been adequately studied for safety.[37] We are learning that the effects of exposure to antibiotics on gut bacteria can persist for months after treatment and sometimes result in permanent disability.

An excellent 2017 review by Zareifopoulos and Panayiotakopoulos suggests that patients should be told of risks including irritability, confusion, encephalopathy, suicidality, psychosis, and mania.[38] In fact, the term *antibiomania* has been coined around the potential for antibiotics to induce manic symptoms. In a recent review, two-thirds of the mania inductions were in male subjects.[39]

The resolution of acute-onset mania with charcoal, which binds foreign toxicants and bacterial by-products in the gut, suggests that these psychiatric risks may be both microbiome dependent and independent.[40] Relatedly, data suggests that there is a dose-dependent risk of new-onset depression; the higher the antibiotic exposure, the higher the risk of depression.[41] In a large case-control study conducted from 1995 to 2013, antibiotic usage was found to precede diagnosis and treatment for depression with recurrent courses of penicillin antibiotics resulting in a two- to five-fold increase in depression diagnosis.

**Vaccines.** It might surprise you to know that vaccines are potential drivers of psychiatric struggles like depression. According to several studies, depression, stress, and dysbiosis can load the gun while vaccines pull the trigger on prolonged inflammatory responses and adverse reactions.[42] On the other hand, some studies indicate that depression and other psychiatric phenomena may result from vaccination effects.[43]

How do you know if you will suffer psychiatric consequences from a routine vaccine such as Gardasil, a booster shot for tetanus, or the annual flu shot? You don't.

Vaccines were designed before we knew about DNA, viruses that contaminate cells used to produce them, the microbiome, or how toxic one chemical can be to one person while leaving another unscathed. One-size-fits-all medicine is no longer appropriate, and we just don't know how to determine who might be at risk for adverse effects ranging from psychiatric conditions to death.[44] For further scientific exploration of vaccines and brain health, you can download a free ebook from kellybroganmd.com.

# Before You Begin the One-Month Reset

Now that you've identified the most prevalent physical conditions that can masquerade as various forms of mental and emotional disorders, you are ready to begin a program, outlined in the next chapter, that will not only eliminate their causes but also reset your body, mind, and soul for lasting wellness. First, however, you might consider exploring some key laboratory tests to establish a baseline and help in assessing whether psychiatric pretenders are masquerading as mental and mood disorders.

The following are my recommended lab markers, which can be ordered through independent, direct-to-consumer labs (see the Resources section of my website for details) or through a trusted clinician.

## B$_{12}$

Blood levels above 600 ng/mL are ideal. An elevated MCV level (above the reference range) and homocysteine can also be functional indicators. The optimal level of homocysteine is between 7 and 10 µMole/L, but when I see a homocysteine level over 8, I recommend supplementing with activated B$_{12}$ (methyl, hydroxy, or adenosylcobalamin) to replenish.

### Thyroid

Optimal values:

- TSH: less than 2 µU/mL
- Free T4: ideally over 1.1 ng/dL
- Free T3 (FT3): ideally over 3.0 pg/mL
- Reverse T3 (RT3): less than a 10:1 ratio RT3:FT3
- TPOAb: less than 4 IU/mL (or near negative according to lab range)
- TgAb: less than 4 IU/mL (or near negative according to lab range)

### Blood sugar

Optimal values:

- Hemoglobin A1C: 4.8 to 5.2 percent
- Fasting glucose: 70 to 85 mg/dL

- Fasting insulin: below 6 µIU/mL

**Gluten and dairy sensitivity**

While many practitioners recommend food allergy and sensitivity testing, in my opinion, the science isn't quite there yet and can often lead to healthy foods avoided and unhealthy foods embraced. My take? Try eliminating the foods you think you may be sensitive to for a period of time and then reintroduce them one at a time and see how your body responds.

## Travel Tips

### Tip #1: Beef Up Your B$_{12}$

Animal foods are the best food sources of vitamin B$_{12}$, including organ meats, grass-fed meat, wild-caught fish, organic poultry, and pasture-raised eggs. Algae and fermented foods may represent promising options for some diligent individuals. Supplementation is often initially helpful, however, especially for people who test low and can monitor their levels.

### Tip #2: Choose a Birth Control Alternative

If you're taking birth control for contraception, own your right to keep Big Pharma out of your bedroom to bring your full vital self to your sexuality and work with your body, not against it. I recommend a non-hormonal IUD, or my personal choice, a body temperature monitor and personal fertility tracker, called the Daysy.[45]

### Tip # 3: Got a Headache? Take Turmeric, Not Tylenol

Now that you know the dangers of Tylenol and other NSAIDs, you'll want to know what to take for headaches and other aches and pains. I recommend turmeric, the yellow root found in curry powder that contains a powerful anti-inflammatory and pain reliever called *curcumin*. This has been used in Ayurvedic and Chinese medicine as a treatment for pain, digestive disorders, and wound healing for centuries. Many studies show the beneficial effects of curcumin: curcumin works as well as ibuprofen to alleviate pain from knee osteoarthritis[46] and PMS.[47]

Next time you have a headache, reach for 1 to 2 grams of curcumin—or even tastier, a turmeric latte.

**Turmeric Latte**

Preparation time: 10 minutes

- Combine 1 cup water with ½ cup organic turmeric powder in a saucepan and heat on low for about 7 minutes, adding more water (up to 1 additional cup) if it becomes too dry.
- Remove from heat and stir in ⅓ cup unrefined organic coconut oil or extra virgin olive oil, and ½ to 1 teaspoon black pepper.
- Store this in a glass container in the fridge.

In the morning:

1. Put 1 teaspoon of paste in a mug.
2. Add a dash of warming spice like cinnamon, cardamom, clove—or all three!
3. Add raw honey (to taste).
4. Pour in about ⅓ cup unsweetened almond, coconut, or hemp milk.
5. Fill the rest of the mug with boiling water and stir.
6. On those days when you need a little more resilience, toss in some sliced garlic if you dare!

༄

## What's Next . . .

In the chapter that follows, you will be given the steps for a one-month lifestyle and dietary Reset protocol that has worked for patients, course participants, and readers alike, to return body and mind to a lived experience of their true selves.

Chapter 6

# A REUNION
# WITH YOUR BODY
# IN ONE MONTH

*Each person is the ultimate authority on his or her bodily
requirements, and . . . the body will reveal its requirements
given sufficient attention and trust.*

— CHARLES EISENSTEIN, *THE YOGA OF EATING*

A felt experience of healing—the *experiential* knowing that your
body has the power to self-regulate and recalibrate—is something
you can achieve in one month by following a protocol I've taken
thousands through in my practice and my online program, Vital
Mind Reset. In this chapter I will show you how to engage that reclamation ritual over a one-month period, so you have a foundation on
a physical level for a transformation that encompasses your mental,
emotional, and spiritual experience.

However, my recommendations for dietary and lifestyle changes
should not be seen as a means to an end, that end being a perfect
and happy life. Rather, the outcome will create a new future as a way
of life, and will begin the loosening of the old ways, the costumes
that no longer fit, and that false "you" who needs to go.

## COMMITTING TO SELF-CARE

It is my belief that healing begins with a reunion with your body—meaning you no longer see yourself as separate from your body but as a whole self—body, mind, and soul. This healing entails a daily commitment to structured self-care as described in this chapter. Through this simple but powerful posture, you feel shifts and changes that you are responsible for (and have not outsourced to pills), and you begin to experience the expansion of your innate power.

Here is what I say to all my patients when they are embarking on my month-long Reset protocol: *You need a month of serious prescription-level commitment to change. ONE MONTH. It's a month of your whole life! It's a blip. The past month flew by so quickly you can barely tell me anything about it, I bet. So stop listening to all those voices haunting you, saying you can't do it. Stop making excuses and look boldly into the eyes of your resistance. Look at it, smile, and push on through.*

When you go all in with this level of commitment, you do it with your heart. And I believe that this intense focus—this uncomfortable level of self-care—is part of the alchemy of transformation. You send your body, mind, and spirit a message, loud and clear, that change is happening. And then, change happens.

A special kind of learning happens when you are feeling the change, feeling the healing. Specifically, you learn what it feels like when you eat food stripped of the addictive push-pull so many of us struggle with. When you quit sugar, alcohol, coffee, wheat, and dairy, you find that you are no longer the irritable, tired, forgetful person you always thought you were. This is valuable *information* you now have about yourself, allowing you to make choices from true informed consent. This type of information comes from what is called *experiential knowing.*

You could read this book and all the studies in it, and love the idea of natural healing, but it won't be until you show yourself your body can heal through a healthy relationship with the natural world that this journey truly becomes *yours.*

The story of Tara, a composite of so many stories I've heard over the years in my practice and online Reset protocol, illustrates the power of making that commitment and gaining experiential knowing.

## TARA'S STORY: EXPERIENTIAL KNOWING LEADS THE WAY

Married with two children and working in advertising, Tara is emblematic of millions of women struggling to make career and motherhood work. Every morning she takes Zoloft (an antidepressant), Synthroid (the most prescribed drug of all to treat an underperforming thyroid), and birth control. If she can't sleep, she'll take the sedative Xanax. She feels like there is a white noise of worry and to-do lists: the general feeling that every day is a race to a finish line while trying to avoid any major collisions or catastrophes along the way. She feels tired, irritable, overweight, achy, and cloudy. Some days, she spends the whole day fantasizing about the glass of wine she'll pour when she gets home. She watches the news and worries about terrorism, outbreaks, public shootings, and politics. This is a lot of what her friends talk about to each other, in a sea of general complaints.

Tara loves her doctor, with whom she's been since early adulthood, and trusts him. Her children are also on medications—her 11-year-old daughter is on Vyvanse for ADHD and her 8-year-old son is on inhalers and oral medications for severe asthma; he carries an EpiPen wherever he goes. Tara spends a lot of time at the pediatrician's office and has to go to the emergency room for various illnesses from cough to fever about three or four times per year.

It would be accurate to say that Tara is just surviving until she dies. She feels a profound sense that this is not how life is meant to be lived. That something is missing. That she is outside looking in, disconnected, and disoriented but doesn't feel like she has any idea how to change. Somehow she ends up learning that there's another way. She books a consultation with me.

From the moment Tara decides to see me as a patient, we embark on a healing journey together. I share with her the very tools we will discuss here. She commits, and she believes. I look her in the eyes and ask with every fiber of my being, *Are you ready?* She is ready.

Through the process of physical healing resulting from her commitment to clean living and meditation, Tara begins to have the *experiential* knowing that her body has the capacity to self-regulate. Long-standing symptoms like fatigue, constipation, hair loss, cloudy thinking, and irregular periods resolve. She is sleeping well and feeling clearer, more hopeful, more connected. In this process, she tapers her medications. About halfway through the process, she begins to develop an uncomfortable awareness. She begins to feel that she needs to change her job and engage her husband in a more conscious connection. She feels the plates moving beneath her.

The fear of change is powerful, but Tara has developed a deep sense of trust in what the universe has in store for her. The emergent symptoms and withdrawal effects of her antidepressant taper have forced her to examine what it is that she is committed to and *why*. Her mantra is *I'm coming home to myself, and this is all part of that process.*

## THE THREE PILLARS: DIET, DETOX, AND STRESS RESPONSE

By the time Tara completed her initial transformation through my Vital Mind Reset protocol, she was drug free with a new career and outlook on life. The three-part support system that enabled Tara to have such amazing results consists of:

- **The dietary pillar.** Heal addictive relationships with wheat, dairy, coffee, alcohol, and sugar by eliminating these ingredients for one month; reset your microbiome by restricting grains, legumes, and white potatoes. Drink lots of filtered water, use natural salt liberally, and enjoy blood sugar–stabilizing fats that taste amazing. After the month, you'll make some mindful reintroductions.

- **The detox pillar.** Clean and detox both your body (external and internal) and your environment. Become an educated product consumer.

- **The stress-response pillar.** Establish a three-minute daily meditation. Pay attention to a regular program of movement and sleep.

In this chapter, I'll take you through these three pillars that form the basis for a self-care program and routine to reset. Then, if you want more step-by-step guidance, you can find more detail in my earlier book, *A Mind of Your Own*, my online Vital Mind Reset protocol, and a slower, more step-by-step healing opportunity in our online membership community, Vital Life Project.

## THE DIETARY PILLAR

My dietary recommendations are rooted in my own health journey reversing Hashimoto's thyroiditis, as well as the years of working with patients and watching them transform through a template that Dr. Nicholas Gonzalez called "the balanced carnivore."

There is no one diet, of course, for everyone, but especially for the parasympathetic-dominant types, there is a good template to explore, and to the chagrin of the more dogmatic yoga and spiritual community, it is an acidic diet notable for its inclusion of red meat, which stimulates the sympathetic system and balances these stressed beings. If this is the right approach, you'll know it. Something deep inside you will say *yes!*

Here is a message from one of my patients, who reluctantly incorporated more red meat into her diet with near immediate results that we would never imagine could be helped by such an intervention. "I started eating red meat daily to address the reactive hypoglycemia and am feeling so much better! I'm a lot less hungry, can fall asleep more easily, and then stay asleep! (I can't believe this works.)"

For years, I have observed that conscious inclusion of red meat into the therapeutic diets of my patients—those coming to me for labels of depression, chronic fatigue, fibromyalgia, ADHD, autoimmunity, and chemical sensitivity—is an essential part of the alchemy of healing. This observation has been extended now to the hundreds who have participated in our online healing program, Vital Mind Reset.

And the science backs it up: In an Australian study entitled "Red Meat Consumption and Mood and Anxiety Disorders," researchers looked at a sample from a cohort of 1,046 women aged 20 to 93 and found that those who ate less than three to four servings of beef or lamb a week were twice as likely to be diagnosed with depression and/or anxiety.[1] Australian meat is by and large grass fed, a highly relevant variable in this type of study. They controlled for variables including the "healthy user bias" as well, finding that demographic and lifestyle differences could not have accounted for the finding.

Nick Gonzalez taught me how we have co-evolved with the environment over millions of years, in different ecological niches. In these different niches, our nervous systems adapted to survive. Our ancestors interacted with the available food, the climate, and the microbes, and their bodies met and yielded to these forces like stone eroding from the waves. Those who survived, over time, had to be designed to complement the environment. From the Eskimos to the Amazonians, the alkaline versus acidic nature of available foods selectively stimulated arms of the autonomic nervous system to perfectly balance a system's native dominance.

There are those who thrive on a low-meat, high–leafy green, and citrus diet, and those who thrive on a high-fat, meat-three-times-a-day regimen. And it turns out that your temperament and bodily habits say a lot about where you fit in this spectrum. Nick's mentor, Dr. William Kelley, elucidated 12 dietary types on a map and also personally and clinically tested hundreds of nutrients for their properties in stimulating the para and sympathetic arms.

Here are three reasons I personally recommend a high-natural fat, no-sugar/no-grain/no-legume, month-long diet that eliminates corn, soy, dairy, and gluten:

1. Blood sugar instability can drag your insulin and cortisol levels around to an extent that impacts your thyroid, sex hormones, and immunity.

2. Low fat or diets that are heavy on the wrong fat (trans, hydrogenated, heated vegetable oils) can compromise your central nervous system's ability to support cell membrane functioning as well as hormone production.

3. Inflammatory foods like gluten and processed cow dairy can also provoke brain-based reactions and immune system dysregulation. For these reasons and more, you deserve a month-long Reset.

This natural approach not only helps you reclaim control of your mind, but it can realign your cravings to become a *primal driver* toward a state of balance. Once the mind-bending junk is removed from your diet, your natural preferences will guide you to choices that are right for you.

Make the commitment—and your whole life will change. It's critical to view this commitment as stepping into your power rather than as an exercise in self-deprivation, renunciation, or limitation. You are turning toward different choices, ones that will bring you closer to a clear understanding of your relationship to your body. On the next page, I'll introduce you to five simple rules to guide you in creating your plan.

## LINDSEY'S STORY: AWAKENING TO A NEW REALITY

Twenty-one-year-old Lindsey struggled with crippling depression, anxiety attacks leading to hyperventilation so severe she would pass out, and a bipolar state of mind that had her going between ego-driven highs and numbing lows. She withdrew herself from family and friends and her relationships suffered.

After medication and therapy both failed, she describes thinking, "This is it. I'm never going to know happiness. I'm just broken." It was at that point when she discovered the one-month Reset program in *A Mind of Your Own* and followed it as if "my life depended on it."

Eight months later, she had this to say: "The one-month program didn't change my life; it gave me a new one. It was as if I'd been wading through mud and something lifted me up to solid ground. It's not like a magic wand was waved and everything turned to sunshine and rainbows. It was rather a clarity. I could see and experience my life without any filter.

"I have awakened into a new reality where I appreciate every smell, touch, taste, sound, and sight I experience. My diet still stays about 80 percent consistent with what is recommended, and I've found what foods trigger what reactions, and am confident in my ability to get back up anytime I find myself slipping."

## FIVE RULES FOR STARTING THE PLAN

### Rule #1: Eliminate processed food

In doing a dietary Reset, you'll first want to wipe the kitchen slate clean of all industrialized foods and go back to an ancestral diet—meat, fish, eggs, vegetables, fruits, nuts, and seeds.

*Processed food* is a somewhat ambiguous term. For our purposes, it means anything in a package that has a long list of ingredients, most of which you would have difficulty pronouncing. Why is this elimination so critical to your success in this program? Below I give details of each kind of processed food you're likely to encounter, with a clinical explanation of why it's important to eliminate it, as well as the effects you are likely to experience:

- **Eliminate refined carbohydrates**

    Why it's important: Refined carbohydrates promote unstable blood sugar, contain residual pesticides, and are made from potentially immune-stimulating grains.

    Effect: Ever notice how that bagel in the morning has you slumping over at your desk by lunch? Eating refined carbohydrates spikes blood sugar and can cause "false energy," i.e., jitteriness, irritability, and lack of focus. The pendulum swings the other way within hours, leaving you with a corresponding crash, often resulting in cloudiness and fatigue. When you're on the roller coaster of these foods, it can feel a lot like anxiety attacks and brain fog—two of the most common psychiatric complaints.

- **Eliminate antigens—casein, gluten, soy, and corn**

    Why it's important: Gluten, soy, and corn are the most hybridized, processed, and genetically modified foods on the planet. Casein-containing dairy products are derived from animals that are fed unnatural diets, confined, and medicated. Then the dairy is homogenized and pasteurized to be rendered a lifeless white substance that can stimulate silent inflammation and chronic intestinal imbalance.

    Effect: Processing of these foods has rendered them unrecognizable to our immune systems. They become vehicles of unwanted information, creating peptides that leak through the gut barrier into the bloodstream, stimulating the brain, digestive, and immune systems in inflammatory and even mind-altering ways.

- **Eliminate sugar**

  Why it's important: Sugar is now concentrated, highly refined, and hidden in everything, causing unhealthy amounts to sneak into your diet, wreaking havoc on blood insulin levels, hormones, and metabolism.

  Effect: In addition to contributing to mood swings, anxiety attacks, and the high/low energy roller coaster, sugar causes changes to your cell membranes, arteries, immune system, hormones, and gut. In short, it weakens the very cells of our body.

---

### Resetter: Kris

Since completing the program, I've noticed how much calmer I am. I have an intense personality and am a little ADHD with anxiety. Getting the gluten/sugar/dairy out of my diet has done wonders for my mood. Less PMS (yet still sensitive), better sleep, no volatility, and I've lost 10 pounds. I have to say the KB Smoothies [See Travel Tip, Chapter 2] are a life changer. If I miss a few days, I feel foggy and forget things, but as soon as I have one or two days I'm back to being clearheaded and have consistent energy throughout the day.

---

## Rule #2: Eat whole foods

Eliminating processed foods leaves a big gap in the Standard American Diet (SAD). What fills the void created when you chuck the cardboard boxes filled with chemicals, pesticides, and GMOs?

- Organic fruits and vegetables
- Clean meats
- Pastured eggs (pastured, not pasteurized)
- Healthy fats such as nuts and seeds

Spices, herbs, and natural seasonings can be used liberally, especially garlic, ginger, and turmeric—all of which are shown to have mood-lifting and anti-inflammatory properties. Some seasoning mixes contain MSG and gluten; avoid them unless you recognize *every* ingredient listed.

Salt is another healthy, vital food that has been corrupted through food industrialization. Throw away your iodized salt canister and buy unprocessed sea salt, or one of the beautiful, natural pink or black salts that boast extra minerals from the earth and sea. Consumption of these highly mineralized salts supports electrolyte balance, hydration, pH balance, and detoxification, among many other healthful effects. In order to get enough iodine, I recommend starting with Atlantic sea vegetables.

## Rule #3: Eat plenty of natural fat

Fat is the most falsely maligned element of the modern diet. While certain types of fat most certainly contribute to health problems, a diet that is high in healthy fats is one in which our hearts and brains truly thrive.

Don't let the bad press about saturated fats fool you either. Saturated fats are critical to cell membrane integrity and brain health. We need all types of fat—as long as they are from high-quality sources, such as these:

- Omega-3 and omega-6 (polyunsaturated) fats: cold water fish, flax oil, grass-fed meat, eggs, nuts, and seeds
- Omega-9s (monounsaturated) fats: olive oil, avocado, almonds, eggs, lard (yes, lard)
- Saturated fats: red palm oil, animal meats, ghee, dark chocolate, coconut oil (remember, fats help with absorption of fat-soluble vitamins D, A, K, and E)

**A note about cooking with oils:** Grass-fed ghee is best for high-heat cooking; coconut oil for medium-heat; olive oil for sauté, low, and no-heat cooking.

## Rule #4: Include probiotics

We are living in a time of awakening around many established cultural beliefs. The tide is turning away from denatured, low-vitality, meals-in-a-box and toward living, wild, ancestral foods.

Our ancestors knew these foods were powerful: all traditional cultures have fermented foods in their diet such as kimchi; lacto-fermented pickles, ginger, carrots, and beets; kefir; and kombucha.

Eating fermented foods protects your gut lining from the overproliferation of species of bacteria that are a harmful byproduct of the SAD diet. This microbial imbalance is suspected to be a factor behind chronic fatigue, skin problems, certain autoimmune conditions, and, yes—depression, brain fog, and other psychiatric conditions.

Research clearly shows positive clinical outcomes being produced by minimal but repeated exposures to probiotic bacteria. I have seen complete reversals of strongly presenting symptoms through dietary change alone. Improvements in mood, blood insulin levels, and markers of inflammation are all shown to result from these changes in how we feed our bodies.

**A note about supplements:** You can take a break from supplements during your one-month Reset to see the full effect of diet alone on your physiology. I especially advocate abstaining from supplements if you are unsure whether or not you should be taking them. If you are invested in and benefiting from your supplement regime, you may choose to keep your same supplements on board, but *do not* take any additional supplements during this Reset. The one exception is the use of digestive enzymes and/or pancreatic enzymes, which may help in the case of significant digestive issues.

## Rule #5: Eat mindfully

Finally, I am going to ask you to make what may be the hardest change of all for many of us: take time to slow down, enjoy, and give thanks for the food you eat. Instead of grabbing a cup of coffee as you run out the door in the morning, I am asking you to sit and eat. Instead of staring at your computer while mindlessly shoveling in your lunch, I am asking you to sit and eat. Rather than eating dinner in front of the television, I am asking you to sit and eat. In fact, I love spiritualist, parenting guru, clinical psychologist, and author Dr. Shefali Tsabary's recommendation of disassociating socializing with eating, taking family dinners off the proverbial table in favor of eating in response to hunger.

As a doctor sometimes working 20 hours in a day, I can't tell you how many times I ate a meal with no memory of what it tasted like or how it felt to go from hungry to nourished. This lack of mindfulness has another side effect: it doesn't prepare our bodies to receive food. In many ways, not being mindful of our meals robs our bodies of the nutrients we *should* be getting from our food.

Our bodies need to build up the digestive fire that converts the nutrients in food into usable calories. This process actually starts when you anticipate a delicious meal that is soon to come. It's called the *cephalic phase* of nutrition, and it refers to your mental and emotional experience of eating that begins before you take the first bite. The response deepens when you smell the aromas of food cooking, and you begin to salivate. These reactions are primal; you don't have to do anything to make your mouth water. Just slow down and pay attention to your food.

I am not going to get metaphysical here, but there is something profound to be said for allowing a feeling of gratitude to radiate throughout your body before you begin your meal. There's a reason why ancient cultures knew to give thanks before eating.

This conscious acknowledgment of the gift and bounty of the earth will prepare you mentally and spiritually to receive the nourishment you are giving yourself. Eating well is a sacred act of self-care; you want to start treating that act with the respect it deserves. And in return, your food will respect and serve you: your health, your vitality, and ultimately, the life you want to live.

## PREPARATION FOR THE RESET DIET: ELIMINATE AND RESTOCK

**Clean up your kitchen.** In the days leading up to your new way of eating, you'll want to take inventory of your kitchen and eliminate items you'll no longer be eating. Your goal is to have a clean, organized pantry with plenty of room for the new items you'll be purchasing this week when you restock.

These are the food products and beverages you are turning away from:

- **Grains:** All of them, including rice, oats, millet, amaranth, corn, sorghum, and grains containing gluten: teff, einkorn, barley, bulgur, couscous, farina, graham flour, kamut, matzo, rye, semolina, spelt, triticale, wheat, wheat germ (quinoa and buckwheat are fine).

- **Dairy and soy:** All dairy, including dairy butter, milk, yogurt, cheese, cream, and ice cream, and soy, including soy milk, cheese, burgers, hot dogs, ice cream, yogurt, soy sauce, and anything that has "soy protein isolate" on the list of ingredients.

- **Legumes:** All bean varieties, lentils, baked beans, peanuts, miso, bean curd, lima beans, bean paste, chickpeas, dal (dahl).

- **Processed food–like items:** All forms of processed flours and sugar, and packaged foods: chips, crackers, cookies, pastries, muffins, pizza dough, cake, doughnuts, sugary snacks, candy, energy bars, ice cream/frozen yogurt/sherbet, jams/jellies/preserves, ketchup, processed cheese spreads, juices, sports drinks, soft drinks/sodas, fried foods, sugar (white and brown), and corn syrup.

- **Beverages:** All but filtered water.

- **Processed oils:** Margarine, vegetable shortening, and commercial brands of cooking oil (soybean, corn, cottonseed, canola, peanut, safflower, grape seed, sunflower, rice bran, and wheat germ oils)—even if they are organic.

**Then restock.** The following items can be consumed liberally. Go organic and local with your whole-food choices wherever possible:

- **Healthy fats:** Extra-virgin olive oil, organic virgin coconut oil, red palm oil, grass-fed and organic or pasture-fed ghee, flax oil, macadamia nut oil, avocado, coconut, olives, nuts and nut butters, lard, tallow, and seeds (flax, sunflower, pumpkin, sesame, chia).

- **Whole fruit and vegetables,** except white potatoes.[2]

- **Animal foods:** Whole pastured eggs; wild fish; shellfish and mollusks; grass-fed meat, fowl, poultry, and pork; wild game.

- **Herbs, seasonings, and condiments:** There are virtually no restrictions on herbs and seasonings so long as they are fresh, organic, and free of dyes and artificial colorings. Toss out your ketchup and any condiment that's laced with gluten, soy, and sugar or that's been processed in a plant with wheat and soy. It's fine to enjoy mustard, horseradish, tapenade, guacamole, and salsa if they are free of processed ingredients.

**Go shopping.** Shop for the foods that you will eat this week. While you are selecting your items, hold in your thoughts a strong belief in these powerful cleansing foods to support you on your journey into vitality. I recommend that you shop at least once per week, so that everything is as fresh as possible.

**Plan your meals.** Now that your kitchen is in order, and your pantry is stocked, you're ready to get started. In Appendix C, you'll find a day's sample meal plan to give you a flavor for the experience. If you need more guidance, there are recipes in my earlier book, *A Mind of Your Own*, and more detailed support through Vital Mind Reset.

Unlike other diets, this one won't ask you to count calories, limit fat intake, or fret over portion sizes. There is no portion control; portion control happens naturally, with you eating until you're satisfied. Pay attention to when you're hungry, as you'll find your appetite shifting over the weeks. The good news is that this type of diet is enormously self-regulating—you won't find yourself overeating, and you'll feel full for several hours before needing another meal.

I have seen individuals from all socioeconomic walks of life complete this one-month nutritional Reset, and while choosing organic, unprocessed food may be costly, there are many creative ways to bring this abundance into your life. It begins with prioritizing, likely in an uncomfortable way, this diet as the single most important medical prescription of your lifetime. In this prioritization, other seeming financial obligations and reflexive expenditures are reorganized, and this investment is duly empowered with the energy of your focused dedication. Sourcing local, especially as a part of cooperatives, shares, and community-supported agriculture can help thread the needle of affordability and accessibility.

And remember that this is just one month. At the end of the month, your diet will be refined for you and by you, and decision making around lifestyle priorities will become so much more streamlined and clear.

Here is what one participant in the Reset protocol from my first book, *A Mind of Your Own*, said about his results:

I'd like to submit to your evidence bank some data regarding the efficacy of your dietary/lifestyle recommendations. Let me preface this by saying I was diagnosed bipolar in 2001 after the first and last manic episode I experienced, but have long believed I am not bipolar; rather, I believe I have been managing early stages of a spiritual crisis.

After 30 days of being gluten, dairy, and sugar free, here are my results:

- Anxiety is gone

- No depressive episodes

- Sleep, while still erratic, is more refreshing

- Dizziness down by 30 percent

- Agoraphobia greatly reduced

- PTSD is seen; regression happens with awareness

- Down 10 pounds in weight

- Swollen glands under arm gone

- More flexibility, practicing yoga again

- Walking more

- Radically improved pain (back, thighs, carpal tunnel, "fibromyalgia")

- Short-term memory/recall improved by 30 to 40 percent

- Less reactive to events

I feel very calm. Having been in survival mode due to extreme child abuse and undergoing 17 years of therapy, the body, at least for me, was the last piece of the puzzle. My therapist considers my growth and healing miraculous. Thank you and many blessings for your commitment to revealing and sharing truth and the tools to implement it.

## WHAT'S THE DEAL WITH CARBS?

Eliminating all carbohydrates from your diet can lead to discomforting side effects and energy deficits for some. When I first kicked my serious sugar habit, I followed a strict ketogenic diet and felt great for about two months. Then I crashed hard. Brain fog, lethargy, low vitality: all symptoms that my thyroid wasn't getting proper dietary support. To restore the balance I needed healthy carbohydrates. That's when I learned about resistant starch.

*Resistant* or "safe" starches are specific carbohydrate foods that actually help restore blood sugar balance. They are fiber-rich carbohydrates that are slowly digested by our gut bacteria, rendering them nondisruptive to blood glucose levels. Unlike simple carbohydrates that break down quickly in the stomach and small intestine, causing blood sugar levels to spike, these carbs are processed in the large intestine, where they remain partially undigested, or *resistant* to digestion. This undigested fiber undergoes fermentation in the gut, encouraging beneficial gut bacteria and contributing to the health of the microbiome and large intestine.

Safe starches are *prebiotic*, providing fermentable fiber that feeds and supports the roughly 100 trillion cells that make up 90 percent of our body mass—the microbes we play host to in our microbiome. Diets that include modest amounts of fermentable fiber are demonstrated to reduce the risks of irritable bowel syndrome, inflammatory bowel disease, cardiovascular disease, and colon cancer.[3] Adding safe starches can also lower triglycerides[4] and improve insulin sensitivity, making them useful in diabetic and prediabetic protocols.[5]

In this one-month dietary protocol, I recommend elimination of grains, dairy, beans, and white potatoes so you can learn your relationship to these powerful foods, not because they are "bad."

This is the slate-clearing phase where you reset your body to a neutral, nonreactive state. As a part of a strict elimination diet designed to rid the body of most known sources of inflammation and allergic response, the one-month Reset is not intended to support the body's energy needs long term. Most individuals, especially women, will need to incorporate more starches into their diet to enjoy optimum energy and focus. The key is to integrate the right kinds of starches so that your now-healthy body ecology can be maintained.

After your one-month Reset, here are some of the safe starches to introduce, one at a time:

- White potatoes, cooked and cooled,* and/or potato starch
- White rice, cooked and cooled*
- Amaranth
- Millet
- Gluten-free oats
- Soaked beans
- Chickpeas

*It's important to note that allowing white rice and potatoes to cool before consumption is what turns these particular starches into resistant starch.

Reintegration of these foods after a dietary Reset should be approached slowly, to see how your body responds to each type of starch. I recommend consuming only one starch at a time, up to three servings in a day, and then waiting for two to three days before trying any others. See how you feel under the influence of each individual starch. Do you have gas, bloating, brain fog, or intense fatigue? Any reactive foods should be eliminated again for 30 days, and then the reintroduction process can be repeated.

## Helpful Tips

- **What to drink: nothing but pure, filtered water over the next 30 days.** Drink half of your body weight in ounces of water daily. If you weigh 150 pounds, that means drinking at least

75 ounces, or about nine glasses (8 ounces each) of pure water (no tap!) per day. No alcohol, coffee, tea, soda, or fruit drinks of any kind. Some may need to wean off caffeinated beverages such as coffee using increasing portions of organic decaf varieties for a week prior to initiating the program. Then it's just water, water, water because all other beverages, including tea, have diuretic effects and replace vital water intake.

- **Go organic, whole food, and local whenever possible.** In the past decade, there's been a huge shift in the variety of foods available at our markets. Get to know your grocers; they can tell you what just came in and where your foods are coming from. Aim for choosing produce that's in season, and be willing to try new foods like fermented vegetables. Go organic or wild whenever possible—choosing quality over cost has incalculable benefits—and prioritize the Dirty Dozen as listed by the Environmental Working Group.

- **Set yourself up to succeed.** Choose a 30-day window to set yourself up to succeed. Consider a time with fewer commitments, minimal to no travel, and a stretch without holidays!

As you are eliminating addictive foods like alcohol, sugar, refined carbs, and dairy, you will have an opportunity to relate to food in a totally different way. You will no longer be at the beck and call of your cravings, using food as reward and punishment and thinking about it all day long. When you eat, it will taste good, satisfy hunger by nourishing you deeply, and keep you feeling stable. Exactly what food is meant to do!

## LISTEN TO YOUR BODY

The most important lesson to learn as you embark on this new way of eating is to begin to listen to your body. It knows what it wants. When you clear the slate of processed foods designed to bait your animal brain into addiction, you begin to guide yourself toward your best diet.

Let's say you feel like a new person after a month of dietary change, but then you eat a bagel—the same bagel you'd been eating for 30-some-odd years—and you develop a headache and can't remember your password at the bank. You have now defined a linear cause-and-effect relationship in what would otherwise be a sea of dots. This new way of eating is about self-education and mindfulness.

As you go through the program, begin to pay attention to your cravings and preferences. How often do you feel like eating red meat? Two to three times per week or every day? Are you craving fruit, or can you take it or leave it? What about greens? Are you eating them just because they are good for you or because you love them? If you just listen to your body, you will begin to fall into your best diet, the diet that most complements your nervous system and balances your physiology.

---

### Resetter: Cassandra

I am at the halfway mark in my Reset and wanted to weigh in because I'm the skeptic of all skeptics—never believed it would work, but it has. I've stuck to the list of foods to embrace and have resisted the urge to grab coffee. Cravings have gone way down and water intake way up. Even with stress from my husband being away for work, I haven't run to junk food or alcohol to cope. I'm also down seven and a half pounds without even focusing on weight loss. The biggest change, though, has come with my cycle. Mood swings are less aggressive than usual, and I have essentially no cramping when usually I feel like my ovaries are killing me from the inside. Heavy days reduced from three to one and a half, making the rest of the days more manageable.

---

## WHAT HAPPENS AFTER?

The only difference between the one-month diet and the diet I recommend after you have completed this protocol is that you can eventually reintroduce certain foods to see whether your unique physiology can tolerate them, such as white rice, white potatoes, grass-fed goat dairy, sprouted gluten-free grains, and beans.

Here's how to reintroduce some of the foods that were sidelined during your month-long Reset:

**Grains, white rice, white potatoes, and beans.** After the 30 days, pick a day to have white potatoes with a meal; boil or steam them and cool them before eating so they are more starch resistant. Eat a big portion and see how you feel. Monitor your system for fatigue, gas, bloating, or brain fog.

After three days, try white rice—make sure it's cooled before eating. At this point, most of my patients experience notable improvement in their microbial ecosystem and these resistant starches are well tolerated. For many, beans that are soaked before cooking can also be well tolerated. If they cause gas or bloating, it's not a problem to live without them. When you introduce them, try one type at a time in a significant quantity (two to three servings in a day) and continue to avoid soy (because of anti-thyroid and anti-pancreas effects).

**Dairy.** Many of my patients do not go back to dairy. If you are curious about incorporating it back into your diet, begin with the forms that are least likely to cause problems (see below), eat it at least two times in one day, and watch for three days. Most patients experience fatigue, gas, bloating, or nausea if tolerance is an issue. Introduce dairy in this order:

1. Fermented goat's/sheep's milk
2. Goat's/sheep's milk cheese
3. Grass-fed cow's butter (low in casein)

I typically do not recommend adding back cow's milk cheese or liquid because of how difficult it can be to source A2-beta casein milk (the type of casein less likely to cause problems) in the United States and because of "silent" inflammatory responses. But if you want to see how you tolerate it, introduce it in this order:

1. Heavy cream
2. Fermented cow's milk
3. Hard cow's milk cheese
4. Cow's milk

Remember that dairy should be raw and grass fed, which may represent a logistical hurdle for those without local agricultural support.[6]

In short, this new way of eating *is* your way of eating now. Make peace with it, embrace the strength and clarity it provides, and know that you are embarking on a new phase of health and vitality that will feel better than any doughnut could ever taste!

## TRUDY'S STORY: FROM DREAM TO REALITY

Trudy knew deep inside that medications couldn't bring her where she needed to go. But what she didn't know was that she had options.

From the age of 19, she was medicated with multiple classes of psychotropics, hospitalized repeatedly—including on locked wards—and diagnosed with bipolar disorder. Because of limited benefit from medication, she ultimately went on disability, gained 130 pounds, and bordered on a diabetes diagnosis. She said she felt like her medications were aging her body from the inside. Ultimately, she was treated with 31 sessions of electroconvulsive therapy (ECT), which provided some relief but left her with chronic memory loss.

Pulled by a sense that there had to be more to life, she started with a single challenge—changing breakfast—and felt better the first day. Daunted by giving up gluten and her own self-doubt around motivation and ability to commit to self-care, she skeptically but earnestly committed to the program.

In one month's time, she described improvements in:

- Sleep
- Energy
- Resilience
- Mood stability
- Engagement in life
- Joy
- Hope

She wrote, "The Reset program has given me back my life . . . I want to enjoy my life, be engaged with it and thriving in it, and finally that dream is a reality." She also shared with our group that during a post-Reset appointment with her psychiatrist, he stated that "it seems like your bipolar disorder was caused by gluten," quite a validation that she isn't, and never was, broken.

## THE DETOX PILLAR

In the past 100 to 150 years, we've done quite a number on this planet. The 100,000-plus chemicals—largely unstudied for human safety—including pesticides, fluoride, and plastics, put quite a demand on our defenses, including our immune system and liver.

Therefore, I encourage you to implement as part of your month-long Reset regimen a cleanup of your immediate home environment as well as the products you use for your personal care. Then I will tell you about two special forms of internal detoxing.

Start with the external stuff, swapping out toxic cleaning supplies, toiletries, beauty products, and cosmetics for natural alternatives. Plan how you'll update any big-ticket household necessities such as mattresses, furniture, and flooring. And bring in some plants such as Gerbera daisies and English ivy to naturally detoxify the air. Place water filters on your sinks and showerheads and invest in a source of filtered drinking and cooking water like glass-bottled spring water or reverse osmosis.

### External Detox: Personal Care Products

If you have already done the work to clean out your pantry of processed, chemical-laden food, you may think you have the upper hand on what's going into your body. But food is not the only thing we digest. The lotions and beauty products we put on our skin are absorbed directly into the blood and lymphatic system, without benefit of the filtration that our food undergoes during the digestive process.[7] The skin's job is to protect us from the harms of the outside world. But what if we are letting the enemy in through the back door?

The FDA does not currently regulate the ingredients in beauty products, except for a few color additives.[8] The only way these chemicals are questioned is when they are injurious to a "sufficient" percentage of the public to merit a class-action lawsuit.

American women are more bombarded by latent chemical exposures than ever before. It's estimated that we come in contact with nearly 200 chemicals a day, according to the Environmental Working Group (EWG).

It's easy to feel a sense of overwhelm when you wake up to this harsh (literally!) reality. But there is some really good news! With just a few changes to your main products—soap, toothpaste, shampoo, and cosmetics—you can immediately stop the exposures you are most frequently in contact with, greatly reducing your overall toxic burden. By finding (or making) clean alternatives, you will take back control and create powerful, long-term benefits.

## Four Toxic Ingredients to Avoid

1.  **Sulfates (such as sodium lauryl sulfate, sodium laureth sulfate; also labeled SLS or SLES).** Found in shampoo, body wash, oral hygiene products, cleansers, makeup, skin care serums, topicals, hair-styling products, hair color. Linked to cellular damage, reproductive disorders, kidney damage, respiratory problems, and skin, lung, and eye irritation.

2.  **Phthalates (dibutyl phthalate, diethyl phthalate, dimethyl phthalate, fragrance, MMP, MEP, MiBP, DMP, DEP, DiBP).** Found in deodorant, antiperspirant, perfumes, fragrances, all hair products, skin cleansers, makeup, moisturizers, lotions, spray tans. Linked to endocrine system disruption, cellular damage, reproductive disorders, birth defects, hormonal changes, early onset puberty, and thyroid abnormalities, and a suspected carcinogen. Phthalates are one of the worst by-products of our plastic dependency, and its effects are cumulative. In March 2004, the Centers for Disease Control (CDC) did a population sampling that found 97 percent of the 2,540 people tested had measurable levels of phthalates in their bodies.[9]

3.  **Triclosan (triclocarban).** Found in sanitizer, antibacterial products, body wash, deodorant, antiperspirant, all hair products, toothpaste, mouthwash, teeth whiteners. Linked to heart disease, heart failure, reproductive disorders,

> hormonal changes, thyroid abnormalities, endocrine system disruption, muscle function disruption, skin irritant.
>
> 4. **Parabens (any form: -paraben, such as methylparaben, propylparaben).** Found in cosmetics, makeup removers, deodorant, antiperspirant, lotions, spray tans, sunscreens, shampoos, cleansers, body wash. Linked to breast cancer, tumors, endocrine system disruption, reproductive disorders, hormonal changes, thyroid abnormalities.

Acting to remove these dangerous chemicals from your personal care routine doesn't have to leave you without a way to shower, shampoo, and shine! There are lots of safe, effective products that you can substitute for your old soap, shampoo, makeup, deodorant, and even hair color. You can check out some of my favorite products (all of which I have personally tested and love, available on my website under "Resources"). EWG's Skin Deep Cosmetic Database is another great resource for checking on your products' safety ratings and finding low-risk alternatives.[10] Or experiment with making your own products. My friends over at Wellness Mama[11] and ireadlabelsforyou.com have curated DIY beauty recipes and go-to products that pass the integrity test.

Reducing your chemical exposures doesn't have to be hard. Focus on those areas where you have control, and make consistent, clean choices.

## Internal Detox

More than a blog-worthy trend, the coffee enema is a healing accelerator. Because our buckets are full to overflowing with toxicant exposures, this methodology drains the bucket, facilitating regeneration and repair. There are many detox practices, including dry brushing, sauna, neti potting, tongue scraping, oil pulling, and more. The coffee enema is most relevant to those with complex illnesses (including autoimmunity, neurological symptoms, severe hormonal imbalance, and chemical sensitivity) and medication exposures. In those cases, I feel strongly that being part of a healing community is necessary and reserve explicit instructions out of respect for Dr. Gonzalez's deep wisdom on the subject. He often said, "Nothing helps the liver clean out faster, more efficiently, or more effectively than coffee enemas."

Since employing coffee enemas with my patients (and family and friends!), my one- to two-year outcomes of transformation and healing have been accelerated to three to six months. Here's what a VMR participant had to say about them:

---

### Resetter: Veronica

Wow. Okay, so . . . coffee enemas. I tried them for the first time today and have to admit that I'm sold. I'm not sure why I ever bothered drinking the stuff when this is possible, lol. It wasn't nearly as complicated as I thought—things went pretty smoothly—and I actually noticed an immediate decrease in some of my symptoms. I was concerned about the caffeine because I've had higher than normal anxiety and didn't want it to make me jittery. However, I actually feel calmer now than before I did it, even though my energy level is up a bit. I wish I hadn't put this off for so long, but I'm excited to see such positive results after just one go. I encourage everyone to give this a try and see how they feel.

---

It may sound like a fad or some dangerous, fringe, New Age health-nut strategy, but the truth is that coffee enemas have a long history, even in conventional medicine. Dr. Gonzalez told me about enemas appearing back in ancient Egyptian texts and showed me a study from 1941 showing coffee enemas were capable of resolving intensive care unit near-terminal shock in several patients.[12] And one Harvard study from the esteemed *New England Journal of Medicine* demonstrated—in 1922—that the use of coffee enemas successfully treated psychosis in hospital inpatients (patients were discharged in two weeks!). Coffee enemas were even in editions of the *Merck Manual* until the 1970s.[13]

Unlike drinking coffee, which suppresses liver function through its stimulation of your fight-or-flight system, taking coffee rectally stimulates a nerve bundle about 12 inches in (don't worry, you have an average of 25 feet of intestines!) that reflexes to the liver for supercharged detox. The liver is your filter, and your own metabolic waste and chemical or medication exposures pass through there en route (through bile flow) to your intestines.[14]

Most of my patients report a near-instant improvement in mood, cognition, energy; eventual resolution of digestive issues, headaches, and allergies; and even radical skin healing. It can be a one-stop shop for accelerating your healing.

For a detox period, daily enemas are most effective along with twice-weekly 15-minute Epsom soda baths, which you can make by adding 1 cup of baking soda and 1 cup of Epsom salts to your bath.

## THE STRESS-RESPONSE PILLAR

For the final pillar of your one-month initiation, managing your stress response, I recommend cultivating a practice of daily meditation.

### Daily Meditation: Kundalini Yoga

---

**Resetter: Vanessa**

My entire life has been about "yielding my rights," and VMR has allowed me to see self-care in a positive, appropriate light. I am astonished at how powerful the Kundalini Yoga/meditations are! Every time I sit down for the 3 minutes, I think, *This isn't going to do anything. This is so hokey*, and 3 minutes, 15 seconds later, my soul is so much lighter. Like, how does this work so well?!? How is it so incredibly effective? And keeping fresh flowers/plants in my room and office—a game changer!

---

My introduction to meditation was through Kundalini Yoga. When I went to a Kundalini Yoga class for the first time, I found it to be incredibly bizarre, complete with chanting, singing '70s-style songs, and repetitive movements that really felt like all pain, no gain. I didn't get it. But through a number of vectors, it became clear that I was destined to learn this particular technology. Now, having been through a teacher training program, I see over and over again the power of Kundalini Yoga–based meditation to restructure the nervous system, and to do it quickly.

It appeals to my more pragmatic sensibilities that Kundalini Yoga is goal oriented. Each meditation ("kriya") is for a purpose and has been handed down from ancient people, crafted for outcomes in real time. The mantras are for the purpose of cultivating vibrational effects in the brain and nervous system. The breath is for accessing the nervous system in ways that we otherwise cannot. It is the art of playing your body like an instrument. It can be harder than it looks, and what's hard for me may not be for you. You can expect the unexpected.

Because I can't help but anchor my interests in data, I was pleased to find a small but compelling literature on Kundalini including a recent article that compared measures of heart rate variability (HRV) in two different types of meditation. The authors describe the importance of this measure, stating: "The human heartbeat is one of the important examples of complex physiologic fluctuations. The neural control of the cardiovascular system exhibits the complex nonlinear behavior. One form of nonlinear behavior is the continual interaction between the sympathetic and parasympathetic nervous activities to control the spontaneous beat to beat dynamics of heart rate."[15]

Using a technique called bispectral analysis, they analyzed changes to heart rate dynamics in two types of meditation and found that, while different, both shifted "phase coupled harmonics" to higher frequencies. This study complements an fMRI study[16] that demonstrated activation of the hippocampus during this technique, and elaborates upon the application of Kundalini Yoga and meditation for psychiatric symptoms, as evidenced by a randomized controlled trial for obsessive-compulsive disorder conducted by my friend David Shannahoff-Khalsa that outshines most if not all industry-funded pharmaceutical trials I have seen.[17]

A wonderful paper entitled "An introduction to Kundalini Yoga meditation techniques that are specific for the treatment of psychiatric disorders" describes specific techniques for indications ranging from anxiety to addiction.[18] Add to this the research by Dr. Dharma

Singh Khalsa and his team, who have elucidated the power of a 12-minute practice called Kirtan Kriya to measurably:

- Reverse memory loss
- Increase energy levels
- Improve sleep quality
- Upregulate positive genes
- Downregulate inflammatory genes
- Reduce stress in patient and caregiver
- Improve psychological and spiritual well-being
- Activate significant anatomical areas of the brain
- Increase telomerase, the rejuvenating enzyme that slows cell aging, by 43 percent, the largest increase ever recorded[19]

Kundalini Yoga is a one-stop shop for mental, physical, and spiritual transformation. It has literally turned me from a neurotic, controlling workaholic into someone who experiences grace, bliss, and a trust in the process so deep that I no longer even relate to "stress." It is, in a word, profound.[20]

---

### Resetter: Mara

I have found the program to be life altering! I feel less anxious and depressed, and as you've said, "*I* is a *me* I haven't met until now!" The meditation part has been the most beneficial for me. I started with 5 minutes every morning and have moved on to the 12-minute Kirtan Kriya. The resonance and finger touching are cathartic, and give me a calmness for the day. My next steps are to further taper my meds and also begin training to become a health coach.

---

## Don't Forget: Movement and Sleep

**Movement.** Often, the desire to move is a side benefit of dietary change and meditation; in other words, it's hard to feel like you have the energetic resources to exercise when your body is preoccupied with managing a swirling storm of inflammation. If you've been sedentary, start with 5 to 10 minutes of burst exercise (30 seconds of maximal effort and 90 seconds of recovery) and work up to 20 minutes, one to three times a week. This can be done any number of ways, such as walking outside and varying your speed and levels of intensity by climbing hills, using classic gym equipment, or watching online videos to perform a routine in the comfort of your home.

Research indicates that you can get similar health benefits from three 10-minute bouts of exercise as you would from a single 30-minute workout. So if you are short on time on any given day, break up your routine into bite-size chunks.

My desire is for everyone to connect with a form of movement that doesn't feel like exercise, but feels like a release, like fun, like pleasure. I started as someone who hated the concept of exercise because I thought it meant going to the gym. Now I dance six days a week as the foundation of my personal health practice and commitment. Specifically, through African dance I have learned from my teacher and friend Kukuwa[21] I work out my entire body while connecting to a lineage and ancestry that speaks to my soul. It's therapy in the highest form.

**Sleep.** In addition to establishing better exercise habits, use this time to focus on your sleep.

It appears that, as ever, there is a bidirectional relationship between insomnia, depression, and inflammation such that insomnia predicts depression risk (by up to 14-fold after a year) with inflammation as a shared pathway.[22] Inflammation itself, from sources like infection, food antigens, stress, and toxicant exposure, may also lead to insomnia.[23]

Now that we appreciate the role of sleep in optimal immune and inflammatory functioning, how do we correct it when it has gone awry?

- **Create a sleep ritual.** Your ritual might include downtime, a warm bath, or whatever you need to do to wind down and signal to your body that it's time for sleep. Rituals work wonders to help you feel primed for slumber.
- **Go to bed and get up at roughly the same time daily no matter what.** I recommend a 9 P.M. bedtime for at least one

week. Take advantage of your natural dip in energy around 8:30 so you don't have to ride a second wind and struggle to get to bed after 10. Also, this timing allows you to take advantage of the 11 P.M. to 1 A.M. slow wave sleep that is the most regenerative.

- **Keep your bedroom quiet, dark, and electronics free.** Use a WiFi outlet timer to automatically turn off your router while you are sleeping, and put your phone to bed in another room to limit your ambient exposure to biologically disruptive electromagnetic fields.

- **Pop the right pills.** We are, in many ways, socially conditioned to seek resolution to what ails us through pills. Reaching for nutraceuticals is a reasonable place to start and a way to help support the body as it reclaims homeostasis—you'll find more recommendations for a variety of conditions in my Natural Medicine Toolkit in Appendix B. Here are two of my favorites that relate to sleep specifically.

**Homeopathic remedies.** Homeopathy is a complex clinical discipline rooted in the energetic effects of microdoses. It is most effective when an experienced provider evaluates the whole person to come up with individualized solutions. Clinical homeopathy gives us some benign tools that can be applied more generically; many of them have effected radical interventions for my most complex patients. Here's a starter guide—take five pellets of these homeopathic remedies before bed:

- Nux vomica 30C for tension, feeling overworked, stimulant use in the day

- Ignatia amara 30C for feelings of distress, emotionality around insomnia

- Kali phosphoricum 30C for nervous fatigue (mental fatigue from demands)

- Ambra grisea 30C for sleepiness that disappears when you lay down

- Arsenicum album 30C for awakening with anxiety between 1 and 3 A.M.

**Botanical herbs** have sophisticated mechanisms that serve to buffer the effects of stress provocation. Examples include magnolia, passionflower, valerian, ashwagandha, and even orally ingested lavender oil, which has shown comparable efficacy to benzodiazepines.[24] These herbs often present together in professional-grade sleep formulas but can also be taken dried and encapsulated or as tinctures.

Here's what one participant who completed the program said.

---

### Resetter: Kevin

I had insomnia at least once a week, which is no longer happening. I was only having an occasional coffee in the morning and had no idea how negatively this small amount of caffeine was affecting my system. Now with the change in my diet, I wake up far more rested and energized, with no need or desire for artificial stimulants.

---

## DOES IT REALLY WORK?

Diet and detox alone are powerful interventions, often yielding results that were out of reach for many taking the route of medication. But what about people who are diagnosed with a serious mental illness? Can they really expect a reversal of their symptoms through these methods? Those with chronic paranoid schizophrenia, for example: Are they likely to benefit from shifting their diets and adopting detox protocols?

I can answer that question with the report of a mother whose 20-year-old son, after spending six years in and out of locked wards in mental institutions, did the dietary program and daily coffee enemas. Her story of supporting him and his achievements is among the most extraordinary I've ever encountered since advocating this program.

## JACK'S STORY: SCHIZOPHRENIA IN CHECK

Joan is a fierce mother who has devoted her life to her son Jack's chronic and debilitating diagnosis of schizophrenia. Now 20, he's spent much of his adult life on locked inpatient units, forcibly restrained, suicidal, actively psychotic, mostly nonverbal, and of course, heavily medicated. He'd been given diagnoses of treatment-resistant schizophrenia, Asperger's syndrome, complex partial seizures, and Tourette's syndrome.

A poster child for the failure of antipsychotic medication, Jack begged his mother to help him with assisted suicide through Dignitas, a Swiss-based nonprofit that arranges for its members, on reasoned request and with medical proof, the possibility of an accompanied suicide. She reports he prayed every night that he would die in his sleep and not have to wake up to face his suffering again.

"It was painful to watch," Joan told me. "I had no life. I couldn't leave the house. If I had to run and get the meds or groceries, he would phone me to tell me he was having hallucinations. I'd come home to find he'd ripped off all his clothes and scratched his skin raw because bugs were crawling all over him. And a man was chasing him to try to kill him. He told me, 'You don't understand what it's like. I have sixteen voices screaming at me, telling me that you'd be better off without me. I have to kill myself,' just unfathomable stuff."

Clearly, nothing was working. After reading *A Mind of Your Own*, Joan told her son that she'd help him end his life if trying one more thing didn't work, and so enrolling together in my online program, they began an intervention of diet and lifestyle change.

I heard from them five weeks after completing the diet and detox elements and learned that they were *both* on their way to reclaiming their health, vitality, and freedom from a system of abuse. Yes, anyone can heal. With the right information, motivation, and readiness, *anyone* can heal, reverse diagnoses, and come off medications safely.

Jack began with diet and daily coffee enemas. In a few weeks, he'd made comprehensive diet changes with elimination of caffeine, dairy, and gluten and drinking filtered water. He continued with daily coffee enemas.

After being on the program for 19 days, Jack asked to go for a drive, and his mother took him out for a three-hour-long trip. Previously, he had not agreed to go anywhere. He began to ask to spend time in surrounding forested areas, which he found soothing, and now goes for walks on a regular basis, including two-and-a-half-hour hikes or taking the dog on one-hour walks.

One year after beginning this intervention, Jack still hears voices, but they are not as loud, commanding, or negative as the old voices he heard. He's ceased to have visual hallucinations, olfactory hallucinations, or paranoia. His physicians have reported that his "schizophrenia appears to be in remission."

Jack's quality of life has improved substantially. He completed almost 500 hours of volunteer work with three different initiatives: organic gardening, recycling, and a palliative care men's group. He goes to the gym three times per week, has given up smoking, and is obtaining a driver's license. Even after the Reset diet, he continues on a caffeine-free, gluten-free and dairy-free diet, and still does the coffee enemas almost every day.

"It's just been totally miraculous," Joan told me. "No one can believe it. I don't know what else to say. It's amazing!"

I couldn't agree more!

## THE BALANCING ACT

As with so many things in life, discovering and establishing a new habit is a balancing act. Even once you've shifted your eating and changed the way you buy, cook, and order food, you'll still have moments when old habits try to emerge. Now that you have the knowledge, I hope you will stay mindful of your body's true needs every day as best you can.

Whenever you feel like you're about to fall off the proverbial wagon, commit to a month-long protocol again. It can be your lifeline to a healthier way of living that supports the vision you have for yourself. In my experience, even two weeks of recommitting to the slate-clearing template can relieve symptoms aggravated by cheats on vacation or at a dinner party.

When we sit in stillness and watch, we can see just what is in store for us. Sometimes challenges are exactly what the doctor ordered. Sometimes tragedy is part of our path; other times, something amazing can turn out to be a colossal burden. In the world of psychiatry, distress is a sign of sickness to be eliminated by consciousness-suppressing drugs instead of a gateway to change, an invitation to look at and fix what might be misaligned or out of balance.

At the beginning of this chapter, I warned that the goal cannot and should not be perfect health and happiness. We are here, right now, having a real embodied experience of this lifetime, walking a spiral path that allows us to continuously awaken to more and more layers of illusion and unconsciousness. The path is rich with strangeness and wonder, and if you are courageous enough, it will be peppered with mystical opportunities to grow and to look deeper into the hurt places that need attention, love, and care . . . and you won't call them problem symptoms any longer. You'll call them invitations to finally, truly be yourself.

Whatever has brought you to this book is something to be grateful for. It's what you needed to raise your awareness and ready yourself to pass over a threshold. May my message and ideas be a gateway to change.

CRObO

## What's Next . . .

In Chapter 7, we will address the process of tapering off any psychotropic medications you may be taking, and how to approach the experience that precedes your inevitable rebirth, a phase I call the Dark Night of the Soul.

Chapter 7

# MOVING BEYOND MEDS AND NAVIGATING THE DARK NIGHT

*They fall, and falling, they're given wings.*

— RUMI

*I acknowledge, with great compassion, that this is a challenging topic for the many individuals who make the difficult decision to begin treatment with psychiatric medication. Tapering off psychiatric medication is a soul calling. It is a choice that you feel magnetized toward and will stop at nothing to pursue. These words are intended to support that rebirth process. Primarily, the approach outlined in this book is intended to fortify you physically so that you do not encounter the many medical consequences of psychiatric medication withdrawal that are documented in the medical literature. The taper process is a marathon of heroic proportions and requires serious commitment and preparation, including compliance with self-care practices, a supportive and transparent dynamic with anyone living in your home, and possibly the cessation of work during recovery. This is not a "business as usual," "do it on the side" endeavor. In fact, I believe it to be a sacred and momentous passage in an adult life that a small but growing number of individuals are engaging in so they might understand what it is to stop running, and to finally feel whole. What follows herein is a discussion of the taper process as a serious decision to be engaged only when it represents the independent choice of an informed individual.*

⋐ ⋑

Every year, millions of people worldwide choose a pharmaceutical approach to treating their symptoms of mood instability, anxiety, insomnia, fatigue, poor concentration, and general disconnection from life. For you, perhaps that choice provided temporary relief from what felt like an unbearable weight. But you might have begun to question that approach when your symptoms persisted or got worse, creating more negative side effects than benefits, many of which I described in Chapter 2. The resultant pharmacological merry-go-round of *try this pill*, then *try that pill* has begun to weaken your faith in a pill-based cure.

For whatever reason, you have reached a point where you feel less aligned with a medication-based relationship to your life experience, and you are wondering, *What's next for me?* You want out, but don't see any clear exit.

Unfortunately, doctors who prescribe these medications rarely develop a long-term plan with their patients. Important questions don't get answered, such as:

- How long should I take this medication?
- Will I eventually stop, and if so, when is the right time?
- What are the correct step-down dosages?
- What tools and support structures will be most helpful during a taper?

In this chapter I will address these concerns so you can properly orient around the courageous act of choosing to live a med-free life, whether that means tapering off your meds or avoiding them in the first place and instead healing the root cause of your symptoms. If you are not currently being prescribed pharmaceuticals, you will find that the information in this chapter provides a depth of informed consent you might not otherwise be given by your doctor.

I will also be reviewing how the most optimal results of tapering come from a balance of the right timing and preparation, careful management of dosage decreases, and strategic support structures during and after the process. But paramount to all of this is you having a mindset and attitude to frame a strong commitment to see it through. This involves an understanding of what I call the Dark Night phase that can accompany the taper process. In this chapter I will show you how to navigate this phase, which can be a psychospiritual birth canal for your transformation into living an awakened life.

## THE SCIENCE BEHIND TAPERING

In my medical training, I was never taught how to taper a patient off prescription drugs. I have no mentors and very few like-minded colleagues who offer medication tapers in the context of a practice dedicated to nonpharmaceutical approaches in every single patient at all times. Most of what I have learned about psychiatric drug withdrawal, I learned from patients and the arduous road of direct clinical experience. As for patients' concerns about becoming "addicted" to psych meds, I was taught in my training to dismiss them and to deny the possibility of protracted withdrawal, it being seen only as evidence of the clear "need" for permanent medication treatment.

Even today, there is little support in the conventional arena for addressing the issue of tapering. As psychiatrist and activist Dr. Peter Breggin has stated,[1] psychiatric drug withdrawal programs are the most urgently needed intervention in the field of psychiatry today. My own experience and training attest to that need.

Why is this? Probably because the field of psychiatry has long been in denial about (or ignorant of) the addictive quality of the drugs being prescribed. Slowly, this is changing. A 2015 review of 23 studies concluded that the term "discontinuation syndrome"—as psychiatry euphemistically labels the months to years of nervous system instability that can result from medication taper—must be abandoned in lieu of the more accurate term *withdrawal*.[2] Withdrawal points to the habit-forming qualities of antidepressants, and classifies them in the same category as Valium and Xanax, and yes, heroin and alcohol.

Further underscoring the addictive qualities of these drugs, another study found that after drug withdrawal, symptoms can occur for up to six weeks, while after psychiatric drug "discontinuation" (still using the older term), persistent physical and mental disorders may persist longer, for more than six weeks.[3] This study provides a handy chart of the horrors that can befall unsuspecting patients, ranging from those who miss a dosage to those who taper carefully. These include everything from general autonomic symptoms like sweating, chills, fatigue and lethargy to visual changes such as blurred vision, cardiovascular changes (vertigo, tachycardia), sensory symptoms (brain zaps, tinnitus, altered states), and neuromuscular symptoms (muscle rigidity, jerkiness, facial numbness, tremors). Mental symptoms include confusion, amnesia, decreased concentration, anxiety, panic, depression, suicidal ideation, impulsiveness, anger, mood swings, and even hallucinations. Finally, sleep and sexual effects include insomnia, premature ejaculation, and genital hypersensitivity.

In a rare instance of clinical documentation of approaches to tapering patients, one study compiled case examples that resulted in varied outcomes.[4] In it, researcher Dr. Jonathan Prousky describes in detail his approach to these complex cases. He supports patients' reframing of their experience of mental illness, their self-care, and a careful dosage schedule that involves decreasing medication and the use of natural support, such as vitamins and botanicals, as well as amino acids like gamma-aminobutyric acid (GABA) and L-theanine.

I am working with clinical volunteers to publish a case series of 15 successfully tapered and vital women who are now liberated from diagnoses and medications, and we are conducting the first randomized, controlled trial of Vital Mind Reset to further broaden the conversation on this topic in the medical arena.

Here's what my online participant Michele had to say about her experience both before and after coming off her meds.

---

### Resetter: Michele

I am celebrating 60-plus days off all psych meds after being on antidepressants for 16 years and believing the lie that there is something wrong with me—specifically, something wrong with my brain chemistry.

Today, I am centered and calm on most days, despite moving through a very painful divorce (a turning point in my life that is quickly transforming into the best thing possible for me to honor and stay true to myself in my new life).

Here is my secret: I was ready to give up my old way of believing, knowing, thinking, and feeling. Quite simply, I was sick and tired of being sick and tired. I had exhausted all efforts in trying to make my old life work, and because my life just wasn't working, I was willing to go to any length to recover my body/mind/soul.

You can recover and reclaim your life! I did it. I'm living proof.

---

## TAPERING: PREPARATION, SUPPORT, AND DOSAGE

Once you become aware of the undisclosed concerns and side effects of long-term treatment with psychiatric meds (see Chapter 2 for more detailed discussion), you may be thinking, *Get me off this stuff! I'm done!*

Not so fast. I have witnessed many cases of the withdrawal experience and would warn against expecting a short time window for successful tapering. I previously referenced a concerning new study published in the U.K. that reveals how current U.K. and U.S. guidelines underestimate the duration of antidepressant withdrawal, pointing out that it is not uncommon for the withdrawal effects to last for several weeks or even months.[5] And when patients were asked directly in an Internet survey, the reported mean for SSRI withdrawal was a whopping 90.5 weeks (that's almost two years).[6]

### Preparation

There is a way to avoid such extended effects by slowing down the dosage decrease, but even before you get to altering your dosage, there's plenty for you to do. In fact, I never recommend tapering without engaging in the one-month protocol outlined in Chapter

6. It serves to drain your bucket before you add the new stress—physical, emotional, and psychospiritual—of a taper. This is done initially by promoting physical resilience in order to bring back a signal of safety to the mind and body. Such a healing effort will often serve to reverse any physiological root cause of what may have led you to medication in the first place (see Chapter 5).

Once a platform of a balanced physiology is in place, the following steps for strategic support should be taken as part of your preparation:

## Strategic Steps for Preparing to Taper

- Engage a qualified health professional (which can include an experienced coach) to guide you, if at all possible. He or she should be available if you need to reach out during the process. (See the Resources section of my website for referrals.)

- Identify your *why*. Connect regularly to the reason you are tapering; for example, "To finally move past my conditioned beliefs about being broken, and to heal my body, free my mind, and reclaim my life."

- Have nonpharmaceutical tools in place to help surf the emergent energy of feeling states.

- Keep a journal to record each day's progress and experience.

- Inform only those you trust to reflect to you your highest potential. This may be a small circle, and that's all the more reason to join a like-minded community now.

- No matter how prepared you are, know that this is a personalized process that unfolds differently for each individual.

## Support

What can you do that is nonpharmaceutical to support yourself as you prepare to taper? Here are some actions you can take before you taper and as you continue during the process:

- **Start training your body to deal with stress.** One of the most powerful ways to send a signal of safety to your nervous system, as well as retrain your response to stress, is through breathwork. Increase your 3-minute practice to 11 minutes or more a day. I love the aforementioned Kirtan Kriya to begin to engage brain-based healing. Also, consider investing in a home biofeedback device like HeartMath's Inner Balance Sensor to learn how to bring your heart, breath, and brain into energetic resonance, unlocking your body's healing mechanisms.[7]

- **Support your nervous system with supplements.** Shoring up with strategic supplements can often help support the body before and during the tapering process. I focus on calming the nervous system during medication tapers. While there is no magic supplement bullet, nutraceuticals with evidence of promoting relaxation of the nervous system and modulation of excitatory brain ports can be helpful. Specifically, supplements that have been identified to buffer the effects of excitatory glutamate are magnesium, zinc, N-acetylcysteine, and phenibut or PharmaGABA.

  I don't always use amino acids as primary therapy, but they can be helpful during a taper because of signals of deficiency that the body may be getting in the wake of medication discontinuation. L-tryptophan and 5-hydroxytryptophan (5-HTP), and L-tyrosine and dL-phenylalanine can be effective support. Inositol, a membrane stabilizer, and herbs like kava kava, lemon balm, holy basil, and lavender can also serve as transitional aids to relieve symptoms of nervous system arousal. Cognitive impairment can be supported with lion's mane extract, micellized phosphatidylcholine, and omega-3 fatty acids. (See the Resources section of my website for trusted online sourcing options.)

- **Begin therapy to heal your childhood wounds.** Because mindset is a major determining factor in this process, trauma and grief work can allow for a vast acceleration. The taper process can trigger fight-or-flight responses that invoke old patterns and bring childhood wounds to the surface. Here is a simple practice I recommend to all of my patients:

When you feel intense emotion (for example, fear, rage, shame), label it and then imagine turning your body toward a small, same-gendered child who is having that feeling. Speak to that child, in your mind or out loud, in a simple, caring way. For example, "Wow, you are so angry! That is a lot for you to feel and you have been feeling this for a long time! I'm so sorry this is so hard." Imagine soothing this child, touching or holding her. This is a simple but powerful way to practice the separation of your adult consciousness from your old primal emotions that have needed your attention, acknowledgment, and love.

To deal with more complex trauma histories, I recommend the work of Dr. Bessel van der Kolk as a powerful complement to this healing journey.[8] He writes in his book *The Body Keeps the Score*, "Trauma causes people to remain stuck in interpreting the present in light of an unchanging past," and recommends modalities such as eye movement desensitization and reprocessing (EMDR), neurofeedback, sensorimotor psychotherapy, and the internal family systems (IFS) approach to healing.

## Dosage

Once you've made the shift in dietary practices as a result of the one-month protocol and have a strategic plan of support, you are ready to begin the actual tapering process, starting with a decrease in your dosage. If you've been treated with medication for longer than two months, tapering may need to be slow, starting with small incremental decreases in medication doses and the use of liquid preparations and compounds when small increments are not available through a conventional pharmacy. Some patients require smaller doses, some longer time intervals, some shorter (i.e., micro daily dose decreases). Some, however, are able to move much more quickly, with even weekly dose decreases. Some patients may even benefit from a "blind taper," in which the clinician knows when the dose is decreased and by what amount but the patient does not; such is the power of the nocebo effect. I have found that my patients are able to taper more rapidly than most, which I attribute to the foundational resilience of a properly conducted Reset.[9]

Of note, tapering is a relatively new approach and concept, and there are clinicians who advocate for a cold turkey discontinuation and support of recovery, not unlike the substance abuse rehab model. At this point, it is unclear whether or not withdrawal symptoms are always mitigated by taper pace, and I have worked with patients who have tapered diligently and slowly and have experienced pro-tracted withdrawal nonetheless. I believe that one's relationship to medication at the time of considering tapering needs to be taken into account. If you believe that you are taking poison because you have awakened to the toxicity of medication and are having adverse effects, you wouldn't taper a poison. You'd stop it and begin the recovery process. If, however, you feel you need time to move into the new mindset of an unmedicated life, a long taper may be exactly what you need. You, as always, already know what's best for you. In the end, I believe that every person can recover, even though the journey can look very different along the way.

## THE DARK NIGHT: TAPERING AS SOUL GROWTH

So you decide to go for it. You do the one-month Reset, reunite with your body, and decide to taper your psychiatric medication. You feel proud when you are at half your dose.

Then something happens. You binged on cookies; lost one, then two, then eight days of meditation; and had a potentially relationship-terminating "discussion" with a family member. Now you are what you used to call *depressed*. Again.

You tell yourself you were an imposter to think you could ever break free. You question all of your gains. You question your ability to get off meds, and you question who you are. *I don't even know who I am or what I'm doing here!* you sob. And you isolate. You've let go of the rope pulling you forward and now it's whipping around in front of you, behind a boat that's getting smaller and smaller in the distance.

This is bad news, right? Not to me. You have entered the "Dark Night of the Soul" phase of your process, a reference to a poem with the same title written by the 16th-century Spanish mystic St. John of the Cross. Author and healer Joseph Aldo gives us some context in words he wrote as a guest blogger for my website: "The Dark Night of the Soul has been referenced by spiritual teachers for ages. It is an inner journey that one is called to undertake at various stages in life, one where the mind's limited perceptions of reality are utterly transformed. This experience can be considered a form of death: the dissolution of an ideal, a rupture in a comfort zone, and the recalibration of a belief system that is no longer valid for the destiny you are here to realize as a conscious, awakened soul."

In more modern terms, when you enter the Dark Night, you are having what Viktor Frankl, renegade psychiatrist, Holocaust survivor, and author of *Man's Search for Meaning*, called an "existential crisis." This beginning point is one of total dissolution, when your entire defense system, your personality, your familiar (though dysfunctional) habits melt into a protoplasmic blob, and you enter a white-out blizzard of disorientation. But because this process is about soul growth, that white-out blizzard is necessary—it is alchemically required—to erase the tracks of your old unconscious programming so you can lay down brand new, more conscious programs.

You may move into dark spaces that bring you to your knees. Or you may not. It's impossible to predict. Most people you know and love will have no idea what you are going through or why, so if you feel separate, alone, and alien, well, it's because you are. We have been taught, as a collective, to suppress, oppress, and repress these experiences in any way possible, but the Dark Night is a process of shedding, of letting go and releasing, not suppression.

At that point, it may be hard to remember that you are an unusually courageous soul doing hero's (heroine's!) work. Of course, it won't feel like that at the time, because the nature of this work is to sit with your own ugly insides. It's learning to love the parts of you that you've been beating up and hiding for years. It's awkward, cringe worthy, and very unsexy. There is no way around it, however, but to go through it.

## FALLING UP: FEEL AND MOVE THROUGH

Moving through the Dark Night, you can feel as if your entire life is in a *free fall*, complete with a sense that you're heading toward inevitable doom. It's not unusual for childlike terror to overcome your formerly adaptive adult faculties, leaving you feeling like your insides are twisted up in your throat, and your mind is screaming, NO!

Most of my patients spend weeks in this state (not months, not years, just weeks). This is a passage that has a beginning, a middle, and an end. And the key to the bounded timing of this process lies in giving it a context that allows for a radical shift in perspective out of victimhood and into meaning. What you might have formerly referred to by the highly charged and largely nonspecific labels of anxiety or depression (*Here it is again! It's back! I knew I was sick and broken!*), you are now being asked to reframe as important missives from deeply buried places of hurt. Simply put, you are being asked to move beyond the struggle with seemingly random and burdensome anxiety, depression, and fatigue . . . to go deeper, to their wise roots, and commit to learning about yourself and shining the light of acceptance on these dark, rejected, tender parts.

There are techniques to navigate the Dark Night that I can and will share with you, but first I want to offer you a context for your experience. Here is a phrase I hope you'll adopt: *falling up.* (You may remember that children's book author and cartoonist Shel Silverstein has a wacky book of this title!)

I like to think of dark and light as signifying the processes of rooting and expansion, rather than as bad and good. In tapering, you are moving down into the darkness, the unknown, in order to solidify your capacity to move up and into the light, into the open. You are falling downward in order to ascend. You are *falling up.*

In falling up, there is meaning. What if this sense of everything disassembling, of disorientation, of confusion, echoed by the constant questioning of *Who am I? What am I doing here?*—What if all that is a part of the deal? Consider that this is how it feels to shed a false and former skin, to have an awakening into your truer self.

The awakening process strips away all the ways you've learned to feel safe in the world, including control, organization, and intellectualized understanding. From those perspectives, you *cannot* direct this process because you'd be doing it from your old programs: those that you are looking to shed. The only understanding you are mercifully offered in this process is that it is *purposeful,* and it is preparing you for future happiness. It's as if you've taken a wrecking ball to your old house and now you're standing in the rubble; for a while, you will wander around in despair, walking through all the places where the old familiar rooms used to be. But there will come a time when you build the new house because the old one is gone, and it's time for a new blueprint!

As you surrender and raise the white flag, this darkness transforms. Joy is right on the other side of pain, and when you let those dark feelings out—scream, journal your ugliest thoughts, dance— you may even find yourself laughing out loud shortly thereafter. Intense emotion always has an energetic arc.

With release comes lightness and laughter because you are finally *feeling* what you've been stuffing down, sometimes for decades. Your feelings need room to *be* before they evolve and move into other states. But you are *feeling,* and that is so much more gratifying than the distracted, low-grade whir of numbness and anxiety that characterizes life as ordinarily experienced. We all need practice in just simply feeling, of receiving and expressing our emotions in a new way: emotions that are ours, coming from inside, not reactions to things happening to us that we must manage or avoid.

It is all of these feelings—sadness, anger, fear, joy—that go into weaving the tapestry of happiness. This is because happiness is an immensely complex emotional state that we have to ready ourselves to inhabit—contrary to the mythos of our culture that dangles the magic pill, the false, quick-fix bait.

It is only through the acceptance of the totality of your feelings—especially the ones you have cut yourself off from—that you can finally feel whole and achieve the long-sought-after sense of okay-ness. There is no pill that will facilitate a gentle arrival into your own skin, enabling you to walk your own mysterious and glorious path in this wild world. To do that, you must surrender to your feelings and let yourself "fall up."

*But ordinarily we do not discover the wisdom of our feelings because we do not let them complete their work; we try to suppress them or discharge them in premature action, not realizing that they are a process of creation which, like birth, begins as a pain and turns into a child.*

— ALAN WATTS

## PAIN AS A CATALYST TO TRANSFORMATION

Today in my practice, I don't write prescriptions for Zoloft, Abilify, Xanax, Ativan, or Lexapro. Instead, I taper my patients off these medications, and in that process they often experience a redefining of who they are relative to who they thought they were. As they come down off meds, they look under dusty beds and in creepy closets, letting waterfalls of tears finally flow.

In many ways, psychiatric medications bind, bandage, and constrict the caterpillar in the chrysalis so the butterfly cannot be born. They arrest the soul and the developmental progress that felt emotions make possible. Your emotions are a part of you. They demand inclusion.

When my patients are in the darkness of their own metamorphosis, and when the struggle is crushing, and fear and hopelessness taunt them like some horrific circus clown, I talk to them as my midwife spoke to me when I was in the transition phase of active labor. I tell them to watch for opportunities to unite with their experience rather than fight it. The way through is to surrender, accept, open, and trust. To know they are encountering exactly what they need in order to pass through it and come out the other side more whole, transformed.

The patients I taper off psychotropics are given the opportunity of a lifetime to pass through a portal to rebirth. Without exception, as we near the final 50 percent of their dose—sometimes a medication they have been taking for more than a decade—the ground begins to shift beneath their feet. They enter into a foreign territory, and they begin to question everything, including their own identity and sense of self. Sources of pain from the physical to the psychological spring up to taunt them and challenge their coping mechanisms.

In the container of our work together, they watch this. They write about it. They share, and they share some more. We watch as skins fall to the ground, one after another, until these travelers are transformed in the crucible of the tapering process. They invariably agree: it is *so* worth it to move through the fear.

For my patients, being on and coming off medication has been a catalyst to awakening: what they needed to wake up to themselves and often, to what it is that they are here to do, what their gift is. It is often quite a departure from the clock they may be punching on Monday mornings. (See Chapter 9 for more on this discussion.) Importantly, they touch what I believe is the antithesis of depression and the goal of my treatment—*gratitude for life.*

## JENICE'S STORY: CONFRONTING THE PAIN

"I can't do it, Dr. Brogan. I just want to die."

Jenice was in her final 2 milligrams of Celexa, a popular antidepressant, when she hit her wall. "I want it to be over. I'm terrified all the time and I feel like I'm not even in my body. The day feels like one long panic attack," she sobbed as she described what it's like to be in the Dark Night.

Jenice's ten-month taper had been physically easeful up until this point, but 15 years of bottled-up fear were bubbling to the surface in the context of escalating physical withdrawal from the medication itself. To complicate things, in the early weeks of her medication treatment, she had experienced an intense, expansive energy (a common effect of antidepressants that garners the additional label of bipolar disorder in 1 out of every 23 patients[10]) that had her fall into an extramarital affair with her husband's best friend. At first the guilt, shame, and confusion of this felt like it would swallow her whole, but over the course of the first year, she was able to put it behind her, the depression now "treated."

Once as she tapered off the final doses of her medication, she encountered long-suppressed feelings and sent me this communication:

> I think I may be in the surrendered stage. I recognize the description of being smashed, that my life is crushed and that it is over. Terror and incredible self-attacks in the guise of tsunami-like waves of judgment from God, from life: I am a terrible person, I am the cause of my own destruction telling myself to give up. Feels like what the mystics have described as purgatory or being in the bardo.
>
> I am sorting as best I can: to surrender to the waves and let their destruction happen, yet not let myself attach to thoughts and try to problem solve them. This is when I get in real trouble. This morning I decided to just watch and be completely still and make no story. At once my mind silenced and there was peace for a while.

We paused her taper to gather more support for her process (practicing Emotional Freedom Technique [EFT] tapping, increased coffee enema frequency, and flower essences), and to let the alchemy of these emerging feelings bring forth its magic. As a result, she decided to come clean with her husband and free herself from her energy-draining secret. Their relationship is richer than ever, and the rest of the taper was a breeze.

Jenice's experience of tapering allowed her to confront pain she had suppressed for years. While her panic attacks may have signaled a call for more medication in a conventional setting, in our process together she found that the drug was in fact restraining her pain and preventing her from recognizing it. She needed to own that pain to transform it, so the panic attacks could finally disappear.

## NAVIGATING YOUR DARK NIGHT: THE ONE BIG LIE

The one big lie that your mind will tell you when you are in that Dark Night is this: *I am never going to feel okay again.* This is the lie that drives people to self-destruction. It is the pole holding up the banner of hopelessness. It is the dark cloud obscuring the sun. This lie drives our fear and activates the masculine survivalist response so that we scramble to do, fix, mitigate, and stem the bleeding in any way possible.

When you're in the Dark Night, the imperative is to simply let it hurt, because *this is what change feels like.* Your personality was your effective defensive structure, so, obviously, your personality is going to fight to stay in place. Your mind is going to scare you away from proceeding, even when there is nowhere to go but forward. And that's because it's about to die. Yes, the false you is crumbling, and the most common sentiment I hear at this stage is *I don't even know who I am anymore.*

These words are the harbinger of transformation and an opportunity to *get real, get well,* and *get free.* It's never too late to drop the mask and become yourself, liberated from the childhood conditioning that is keeping your fear at a white noise hum in the background of your seemingly normal life.

Hold your vision of what freedom feels like to you. What I hear over and over again from the people I help is that it feels like finally coming home to yourself.

Remember these guidelines:

- **When you don't know what to do, wait until you do.** We are used to making decisions from our cognition. Pros and cons, better now than never, better safe than sorry. In these times of your life, however, when you feel the ground moving beneath your feet, proceed in a different way. You will know when you have to make a move and what it should be because it won't feel like a choice; rather, you'll see that the only way forward is through. Ending a relationship, quitting a job, confronting a family member, sharing a long-held secret: you are able to do what's necessary. This is what it feels like to make decisions from your intuition.

- **Ask for prayer.** In your Dark Night, ask for help, even for someone to pray for you. In my most recent struggle, I had three altars burning for me around the country. And I asked five other friends to pray for me. And not just in the colloquial oh yeah I'll send you good vibes sense: in the real, focused, intentionality sense. In fact, data on remote healing is pretty remarkable, demonstrating improved healing even when people don't know they are being prayed for.[11] Ask them to pray for an easeful transition, for spiritual support, or for what is in your best and highest to manifest. Ask them to hold you in love.

- **Safety mantra.** There may be whole days during which you feel like you are going to disintegrate from worry, unease, and deep discomfort in your own skin. Pick a safety mantra. Mine has been simple: you are okay. Literally, that's it. I would say that hundreds of times a day during the worst of it. You could choose I am loved. This will end. I have everything I need. I will only experience exactly what I can handle. Or anything you wish you could hear whispered from on high. Whisper it to yourself . . . a lot.

- **Make room to fall apart.** The process of coming off psychiatric medication is a major, courageous leap into the wild unknown of the human experience. It is a rebirthing that deserves all the love, compassion, and home-cooked meals delivered that a baby's birth would garner. Let your spouse, your roommate, your friends, your mom know that there may be days when you cannot do what you would otherwise do. This process is precious and cannot be treated like business as usual. It is certainly not always the case, but time away from work in the form of a medical leave may be necessary. Trust me: in my own Dark Night, I never missed a day of work, so I know how terrifying it can be to feel your most identifying tether to your "worthy" self is threatened. Eventually, your relationship to your job will come under the harsh light of examination, even if it isn't during the taper process itself, so the more room you can proactively make for the seriousness of this juncture in your life, the less protracted your process may be.

- **Anchor your soul in your body.** Many believe, and I have experienced, that the soul may want to leave the body during these alchemical transitions. It is a kind of dissociation. (In fact, there's a flower remedy specifically for this: clematis.) Get back into your body through sensuality. Place your hand over your genitals and feel for the pulse. Turn on music that feels like your mood. Move the energy through. Take a bath. Get a massage. Make love or self-pleasure. Often these things will feel like the last choice on your list of possibilities, but that's your fear speaking. Let your soul know that your body can hold it.

- **Accept your struggle.** Remember that you chose to give yourself the opportunity to taper. You are choosing to reclaim yourself. You are, perhaps, the chosen one in a lineage of patterned trauma and unconscious programs to finally break the cycle. Work of this magnitude comes with challenges. There is a tremendous payoff for owning your struggle, turning toward your darkness, and accepting all aspects of yourself: relief, a special kind of freedom. Yes, it's possible for you to feel more like yourself even if you are also a hot mess. It's possible that people will feel closer to you and love you more, even if you aren't what you imagine they want you to be. But you have to take responsibility and own this vulnerability. Be with your struggles; do the field research on them. And give up all hope of controlling this process. The day you do, the shift will happen.

- **Cultivate self-compassion.** Self-compassion is not the same as making excuses for yourself, babying yourself, or lowering the bar. Rather, it is about understanding the tenderness that motivates your stuck behavior, your rigidity, your negativity. It's about looking beneath your habits of control, self-criticism, and layers of victimization and learning more about the hurt that these behaviors are (trying to) protect.

  Beam love and soul-acceptance to these parts of you, because they are asking for your attention and have been for a long time. Let that child out of the locked room and give her a hug. She only ever knew how to scream, sulk, and kick to get your love. She's had to pretend she's in charge all this time, but now that you are finally here as a conscious adult, she can just be her sweet little innocent kid self again.

- **Find meaning in every experience that comes your way.** This is your ticket to freedom. To find meaning is receiving and engaging with curiosity at the same time. In fact, this is the fundamental difference between medicated consciousness and medicine-less consciousness.

  Let go of fighting or resisting whatever feels outside of your control, and play with the idea of saying, *I don't know, but I'm sure there's something in here for me.* Psychiatry wants you to live in a meaningless world, but the emergence of quantum physics and the consciousness movement are asking you to break out of the cage you're in. You can do it, and all it takes is a curious attitude toward your hardship.

## THE TERROR OF THE CHILDSELF

The kind of change we are looking at in the awakening process is big; it involves self-reclamation and integration. You are literally recollecting parts of your soul that fled during points of trauma in your early life. The pain of that fragmentation is so immense that you have developed an incredible infrastructure of defenses to keep from feeling it. And . . . it has worked! Sometimes for many decades! But, there comes a point—often between the ages of 30 and 45—when we recognize that the mask is slipping, and our authentic, whole self is ready to emerge. This emergence involves turning toward the part of yourself that society, your parents, and that internalized inner critic have taught you to hate—the shameful, lazy, weak, stupid, incompetent, ugly loser inside that exists behind the mask, for each and every one of us. It is your arrested childself, your childhood pain and programmed beliefs, locked away long ago and existing now only as your shadow, now being invited into the light by your adult consciousness.

## TANIA'S STORY: TERRORIZED BY HER CHILDSELF

Tania had been in the Dark Night for about four months. As she finalized her divorce from Zoloft after 16 years, the final 10 mg were spiritually decimating. Not physically, thanks to her compliance and commitment to the one-month Reset protocol, but psychologically, emotionally, and existentially.

Tania moved through a period of tears that fell so consistently that I don't think I saw her cheeks dry for eight weeks straight. Then came rage that led this formerly placid lake of a woman to kick furniture and punch pillows. Then came the big oceanic well of childhood pain that was so intense that it left her feeling disconnected, numb, flat, and apart with her heart on lockdown. During this time, she didn't shower, she didn't do the dishes, her inbox was a runaway pileup, and she stopped being able to interact with old friends and family. She felt suicidal and terrified.

Tania's terror is the terror of her childself. Fear this big is what we experience as children. It's life-or-death fear. It's so big that we build complex patterns of behavior around attempts to never feel it again. Those complex patterns become our personalities, and we live thinking that we are defined by these patterns. But what happens when your entire life is built around a personality that is simply an adaptation to feelings of being unsafe and inadequate?

Tania was given the opportunity to tease apart her childself (childhood pain and programmed beliefs) from her adult consciousness, and to finally become an emancipated woman free to create her life, drawing from near infinite reserves of quantum possibility.

I often use this analogy with patients: You—the adult you—are driving your car. Your childself is in the car seat in the back, screaming and crying and telling you TURN LEFT! GO FASTER! NO, NOT LIKE THAT! As you awaken, you are finally breaking the spell and recognizing the fact that you are driving the car, and you know exactly where you're going and how to get there. You turn to your childself in the backseat and you say, "I see you, sweetie. I love you so much. Mama/Papa is here now and I'm driving the car. Everything is okay."

With Tania, our primary therapeutic interventions during this time included this visualization, repeated many times a day, and further soothing her nervous system with time grounding and walking around in nature, a weighted blanket to rest in bed with, longer duration meditation, and flower remedies.

This type of visualization, done even hundreds of times in a day, can help generate an awareness of unprocessed emotions from childhood. It holds the potential for a mindful adult consciousness to be born from these emotions' intense need to be witnessed and felt as real. In many ways, the emotional challenges of the taper (which are also physiologic, in that they stem from an activated fight-or-flight response) are the opportunity of a lifetime to develop intimacy with that childself, so that when she gets activated in the future, she is recognized and consciously acknowledged, her needs calmly represented to the world in an adult way.

---

### Resetter: Sue

Living in denial is such a powerful thing—I did it for much of my adult life. Life was just. So. Hard. Every single day was a brutal struggle, even though externally I had an amazing life. I bought into what others thought of me, including the hordes of doctors who told me I was "mentally ill," who put me on drugs I was deathly allergic to. I bought into the tape in my head that I wasn't good enough.

It was only by coming to the end of my life that a new life opened up for me, and it was only by facing the worst pain and demons I have ever encountered that I broke free to be me. I didn't know I was imprisoned so badly until I was free—but I can look back now and see the chains that bound me for so long. Always, there was a tiny voice inside that kept saying, *Life shouldn't be this hard.* I kept listening to that voice as it got louder and louder, and kept following it to reach the Light, even though at first I didn't see it at all. I just kept reaching for the Light and the Light was there, waiting for me to bask in its glow.

---

## DARKEST BEFORE DAWN: INSOMNIA AND SUICIDE

Ask anyone who has had the courage to give themselves a psychiatric medication–free chance at life, and they will likely tell you about their battle with insomnia that led them to suicidal ideation during the Dark Night of the withdrawal process.

## Insomnia

There is the apprehension that sets in the moment your body hits the bed—here we go again—like some Sisyphean task that never works but *must* be engaged. There's waking in the middle of the night, and then if a few hours are mercifully granted toward the early morning, there's waking in the morning to acute anxiety like a machete being held to your neck.

Like so much in life, there are multiple narratives operating here.

First, antidepressants mess with your sleep. It makes sense that coming off antidepressants would require a recalibration from the disturbance to sleep that these meds induce. According to one study, effects of antidepressant drugs can include increased sleep onset latency and/or increased awakening, leading to an overall decrease in sleep efficiency. Furthermore, the same drugs can suppress REM sleep and change the frequency and intensity of dreaming, with the occurrence of these symptoms on discontinuation.[12]

Another factor is that tapering off meds is a stressor on the body. When your body has adapted to the complex stimulus of a psychiatric medication, even slow tapering can set off alarm bells. This kind of acute stress can drive immune imbalance, so you become sick more easily and autoimmune illnesses flare. It can also induce functional impairment in the thyroid so your neurologic health, energy reserves, and metabolism are taxed. And then there's the effect of the stress-response hormone cortisol on your blood sugar, which can lead to middle-of-the-night waking. It's a difficult process, all in the service of detoxification and regaining homeostasis.

The first two factors make good physiologic sense, but a third point is the one that most informs my counsel when I sit with women who are in the thick of it: insomnia is a form of spiritual challenge. As I watch people come off these medications, I watch them being reborn, and it strikes me as eminently possible, then, that for some, insomnia is a built-in part of the initiation process.

Insomnia is, in fact, a direct portal to the alchemy of forced surrender. Insomnia pushes people to their absolute edge, but rarely over it. This may be because we have assigned sleep a special value in the Western world—it equates to our productivity (good, solid sleep equals better performance), which equates to our value—and if sleep is threatened, we feel the fear on an existential level. Breakthroughs happen when we turn toward our mind and say, *Enough. I give up. I don't care. And I'm not listening.* When we surrender.

Here's what I tell my patients if they hit patches of insomnia in their journey off meds:

- **Accept it.** This is the cardinal rule. Say yes when you want to say no. Not yes, like I love this! But yes, this is, in fact, happening. No worries. No judgment. Only radical acceptance.

- **Get creative.** When creatives experience insomnia, it's often because something incredible can't wait to be born from them. So use this strange window in your life—yes, in the middle of the night!—to try out something audacious. Write stories. Paint pictures. Choreograph dances. You might find that some important insights await you in the fertile hours of this sleepless space.

- **Engage a bedtime ritual.** Make a ritual around your bedtime, consisting of pleasurable, relaxing activities. I recommend a 9 P.M. bedtime during your taper experience. Before, take an Epsom salt bath, diffuse essential oils, drink a Sleepytime herbal tea, play some chill music, or light some candles.

- **Double down on self-care.** I never taper psychiatric medication without the month-long protocol, but even after your Reset, you'll need to commit each day to meditating, detoxing, and eliminating all processed foods. Cut out the refined sugar, alcohol, and coffee for a less bumpy journey.

Thus far, I have never had a single patient develop *permanent* insomnia. Every single one of the women I work with moves through this phase. It's why I have come to believe that on a bedrock of high-level self-care, insomnia can be a spiritual challenge that can actually serve to liberate you further if you choose to work with it rather than fight it.

## Suicide

We have been conditioned to look upon the tender topic of suicide with horror. Perhaps because it represents a failure of our varied systems of control. Perhaps because we are, collectively, far from being at peace with the complexities of death as a part of the human experience. Perhaps because we have to pretend that we have never personally felt anything like suicidality in order to maintain the illusion that the experience of suicidality is pathological.

Suicidality is not one thing. It is not a symptom of genetic illness. It is not rare. And it is not simply a desire to end one's life.

In college at MIT, I worked a volunteer suicide hotline called Nightline and spent many nights on the phone with people on the brink. I learned that suicidal thoughts *can* be a desire to disappear, to not be instead of being. They can be a crisis of faith and a perception that everything is terminally wrong. They can be a deep grappling with whether the universe is fundamentally a benevolent or a hostile place. They can be the stuck belief that things will always be exactly as they are now.

I believe suicidality to be an irrepressible expression of the urgency for change that must be met with the promise of such change being possible. These feelings express the need for deep transformation that feels like a rebirth, replete with the labor pains and expressions of anguish and overwhelm. They are a scream that says, *This way of being, of living, cannot go on one second longer!!!*

## Suicidality as a Symptom of Awakening

"I know that you have helped a lot of people, but I just can't do it. I'm done. I have nothing, my life has been struggle and suffering, and I need this to be over."

And she meant it. Sonia was six months past her last dose of Effexor—a medication she had been on since she was 15. She was now 42.

At any given time, about 30 percent of my patients are feeling hopelessness descend and actively contemplating suicide. They know that I am comfortable with this. They know that I never have called 911. Never put them on a patronizing suicide watch. Never drawn up some promissory note–type contract. I have never implied for one second that they don't have what it takes to move through this. They know that I am not scared of them or their feelings. Rather, I perceive that something in them needs to die in order for them to be reborn, and that this is their raising of the white flag. This surrender is the end of the end and the beginning of the beginning, if only we let the pain come up, come out, and leave. And it does. It moves. It changes. And often, what comes in its wake is exactly the kind of shift that could never have been prescribed, taught, or suggested. It's deep spiritual growth.

In the taper process with patients, I tell them that I am here to help support their body's stress resilience and to offer them a medication taper as free as possible from rashes, hair loss, menstrual abnormalities, electric shocks, body pain, and the myriad bodily signs of psychotropic withdrawal. But I am not here to make it easy or even tolerable on a psycho-emotional level. This is because I know that transformation is a necessary part of the alchemy of a successful taper. The part of them that believed in medication needs to be shed. But that part rarely goes quietly. Transformation requires the death of an old self. Of old beliefs. Of old forms of security and identity. Transformation is disorienting and even terrifying.

That's why you won't hear me say things like *Do the best you can with the diet.* I say instead, *Do the diet because I know you can exercise your power of choice in service of your health.* Many have never had their full potential reflected back to them, only being coddled in their victimhood as an indirect affirmation of their felt inadequacy and brokenness.

In my vast experience in this clinical realm, I have witnessed that dangling the option of a return to meds creates a fracturing for many people who otherwise are working with a deep desire to move beyond psychiatry. If this option is presented as "equally powerful," there is the dissonance around new and old beliefs, and there is a setup for experiences of self-shaming, defensiveness, and projection of judgment onto others. If we collectively hold that walking through the fire is possible, we create a space for honoring and celebrating *that* choice, whenever it feels available.

It is my belief that the darkness that comes with tapering shows a part of you that needs love and integration. It needs to be felt so it can finally move through, with your adult consciousness soothing that childhood injury and releasing the pain of pretending that it was never there.

## Help in the Moment of Crisis

If you find yourself in the dark hole of suicidal thoughts, here are some ways you can "fall up" into the light:

- **See the light at the end.** Acknowledge that your desire to commit suicide is part of your experience of self-healing and transformation. Focus on how moving through the portal of change can lead you to a life so much more incredible than your frightened mind can show you in this moment.

- **Avoid fearful people.** When you are in crisis, it helps to be held in the light of possibility by those surrounding you. Avoid people who marinate in worry and concern and who might resort to reflexive interventions like recruiting the authorities, even if they are your most dearly loved ones.

- **Ask someone to simply listen.** Many who are suicidal struggle with a sense of deep shame; you feel wrong inside, perhaps permanently. An unexpected antidote to that feeling is simply having your reality received by another. Being heard is empowering because through another you can experience that your ugliest truth is not too much. They can handle it, and in doing so, reflect back to you that what you're feeling is bearable.

- **Give a context to your experience.** Symbols are more powerful than words and can evoke an experience of growth and change, such as a caterpillar that feels disoriented in the dark before it has to squeeze out of the tight hole in its chrysalis to be reborn. Keep such images around for reference in times of suicidal thoughts.

- **Inquire to find meaning.** Get out your journal and write to answer these questions: *What do you know you need to let go of? What's not working? What programs, beliefs, and voices are criticizing you?* With this insight, can you turn toward the pain and personify it as your small, hurt, wounded childself? Can you sit with how intense that pain is in order to understand, deeply, how and why you might have developed all these complex patterns of avoidance?

- **Experience yourself as a wounded healer.** This may not appeal to everyone, but it certainly has helped me in my darker moments. When I've been at the brink, I've taken great solace in knowing that by simply experiencing my own pain, I'll be able to help others in the future. The gift is that you are forever deeply connected to others who visit that place you were in. You become a *wounded healer.*

- **Help another.** You would think that when your cup is empty, you can't give. Through the Vital Mind Reset community, I've witnessed that those who are in the depths of a dark spiral and reach out to another to help them, to volunteer, or to otherwise give of themselves are rewarded with the felt experience of their own inner light. This connecting gesture moves them beyond the echo chamber of their own self-focused process and breaks open the illusion of separateness. It can be powerfully healing.

## ROSE'S STORY: STAY COMMITTED

Rose came to see me after having begun the process of discontinuing multiple psychiatric meds and was well into a lengthy and complicated period of withdrawal. She told me that it took her fierce commitment to make it through the taper process, and she described the tools she used for support.

"In 1992, when I was twenty-five, I got depressed and was suicidal," she reported. "Prozac was big, so I tried it, but it didn't help at all. I got stuck in the cycle of trying new meds and going on different therapies, all kinds of self-help programs." Over the next 25 years,

Rose convinced herself that the meds were helping, even though she was continually suicidal and had to be hospitalized several times.

Then, when she turned 50, Rose started questioning: *Do I want to continue this road of being depressed and suicidal every day or do I want to try something else?*

At the time, she was prescribed the antibiotic Cipro for her acne rosacea and had a severe reaction. "I ended up in bed for four months, unable to walk," she said. "While I was lying there, I looked at my bottle of meds and thought, *If Cipro could make me so sick, then what are these meds doing to me over time?* It was a huge wake-up call. I read Robert Whitaker's *Anatomy of an Epidemic,* and that was it! Before I had finished half the book, I began tapering."

Rose was shocked at how painful it was to come off two antidepressants and anti-anxiety medication. For the first 15 months of her taper, she was in bed for about 70 percent of the time, experiencing feelings of being electrocuted, burning in her GI tract, bloating, fear, and volatile moods. When I saw her, she had an underactive thyroid and pain in her legs and feet that came up in waves of intensity. She also complained of constipation, food and supplement sensitivity, fatigue, weakness, weight gain, rosacea, muscle burning, and cognitive symptoms such as rapid circular thoughts, poor memory, brain fog, and poor concentration. She told me she believed that many of these problems were the result of 25 years of medication use.

Two things worked for her that kept her going. First was an unyielding attitude: "I developed a 'no quit' attitude, telling myself, *There is no going back. I don't care how crappy I feel. I am not going to take any pharmaceutical to make me feel better.* I was offered all kinds of 'help,' Lyrica, gabapentin, but I stayed on track and refused the meds. I was totally committed. I had faith that it was going to get better, it was going to pass."

The second thing that worked for Rose was going on a nutrient-dense, super clean diet. "No gluten or dairy, which is the reason why I did not have one single day of depression after I got off the meds," she told me. "If I slipped off the diet, I'd get a sudden feeling of doom. The sugar/gluten combo was the worst." Rose also learned to detox, including body brushing and coffee enemas, which she started four months into her withdrawal and which helped with pain and getting things moving. I introduced her to Kundalini Yoga, and the breathing exercises helped her greatly with her cognitive functioning.

Now pharma free, Rose reports enjoying her life in ways she hasn't in more than 25 years. "My life now is so beautiful that some days, I'm overwhelmed by simple things," she said. "My sister sent me an e-mail, saying *I miss you so much*, and it brought me to tears. I now feel connected to the littlest thing, and it's so amazing."

To anyone who looks at what it takes to go through tapering off meds and feels intimidated or overwhelmed, Rose asks, "What do you have to lose?" For anyone who is in the tapering process and feeling overwhelmed or hopeless, she offers these words: "Have hope, because everything is going to be okay. Just as I did, you are going to come out of this, and when you do, you'll see the world in a beautiful new way."

## MORE SUPPORT WHEN TAPERING: PRE-DAWN MEDITATION

I studied the physiologic benefits of meditation for years before I was convinced that it was as powerful an intervention as nutrition, movement, and detox, if not more powerful. The Benson-Henry Institute for Mind Body Medicine has been amassing before-and-after studies for four decades. I knew all of this, yet I too didn't commit to a daily practice.

It wasn't until Dr. Nicholas Gonzalez died suddenly that out of sheer desperation, agony, and grief I got on my knees and began to meditate. Because I had already been drawn to the Kundalini Yoga community, I knew that my efforts would be amplified if I pulled my weary self out of bed before dawn. They call it *sadhana*, or daily practice, but there is a strong recommendation for it to occur in the ambrosial hours (*Amrit Velā*) of the morning. In fact, I observed that there wasn't a Kundalini teacher who didn't swear by the existential forklift that *sadhana* represents.

So I set my alarm for 5:30 A.M. and vowed not to change it, no matter what. I would use my power of choice to move through the barrage of negotiating voices every morning. It was two months before my entire outlook on life, relationship to my own body, and spiritual dynamism in the world completely changed. I was literally rewired in those two months. I went from a controlling and hyper-vigilant stress addict to someone who knows deeply what it is to feel calm at the center of it all. Today, I no longer experience stress because I feel, inside me, that everything is okay.

And I'm not alone. Daily practitioners sit in humble awe at how their lives begin to take on a magic carpet ride effect: people and information delivered to them in perfect synchronicity, opportunities surfacing effortlessly, radiant health, and access to being in the flow rather than hanging on by their fingernails.

If you are ready for growth, healing, and transformation, do a pre-dawn meditation every single day. You might think that someone in the throes of the Dark Night can't handle one more stressful thing like getting up early to meditate. But because I relate to the *adult consciousness* of each and every patient I work with, I remind them that they always have their will to choose and the power to commit their mental energy toward self-care. Desperation is a powerful motivator, and these are the patients who really derive change from this practice.

With a pre-dawn meditation, you enter a meditative state during a critical neuroendocrine shift in your daily cycle. This has anti-aging effects as well as hormonal benefits, and it sends psychospiritual signals of calm to your system.

In addition, waking before dawn puts you in alignment with evolutionary patterns of wakefulness. We were meant to awaken in the dark. Contrary to the assumption that we naturally rouse with the light, if you consistently go to bed before 10 P.M. (essential for healing!), you will begin to naturally wake up around 5 A.M. or even a bit earlier. In my research, I have learned that the coldest time of the night is about 40 minutes before dawn, and that *this* is when our ancestors (and modern-day aboriginal people) commenced morning rituals.[13]

When we open our eyes in the morning, we should, quite literally, begin weeping with awe and joy that we get to have one more day on this magical planet in this mysterious life adventure. Instead, our minds, like a lighthouse, search for what we have to freak out about. Undo this freak-out, even in a few minutes, and send a different signal to your nervous and endocrine systems. Our stress hormone, cortisol, rises between 4 and 6 A.M. If you can be in an intentionally meditative state during that window, you set the template for your reactivity for the rest of the day.

If you start your day this way, you've already won even before you leave the house. You have set your intention to be your highest self, to push through resistance, to reclaim balance. You can carry this in your pocket all day like a precious gem. It will become an irresistible impulse over time.

## Your Daily Pre-Dawn Practice

### Prepare:

- **Go to bed before 9 P.M.** Stop doing work late into the night (this was a hard one for me, but my productivity has skyrocketed since I stopped working at night!) and stop watching TV. Just go. To. Bed.

- **Set your alarm** for no later than 6 A.M. No snoozing. Sit up in bed right when it goes off. It hurts. I know. But it's really only for about 5 minutes, and then you will ease into your practice and feel the quiet peace of being awake when no one else is.

- **Create space** for your practice. Use a special mat or blanket. Light a candle or burn some sage. Anoint yourself with an essential oil.

### Meditate:

Choose a 3- to 11-minute kriya or meditation, ideally one that you will commit to for 40 days. You can start with just 3 minutes. Here is a favorite of mine called Meditation to Act, Don't React that can be done for 3 minutes to start; you can work up to 11 minutes.

- **Posture:** Sit in Easy Pose with your spine straight, chin in, and chest lifted. Bend your elbows and lift your forearms so that the elbows are not resting on the ribs. From elbow to fingertips, the forearms are at a 45-degree angle forward. The hands are positioned so that the thumb is touching the tip of the Jupiter (index) finger.

- **Eyes:** Close the eyes.
- **Breath:** Inhale deeply through puckered lips with a whistle (3 to 4 seconds), hold the breath (3 to 4 seconds), and cannon fire the exhalation out through the mouth. (Cannon Breath is a powerful exhalation from the navel point through the mouth. The cheeks are firm and the pressure of the breath passes over the tongue and out the mouth, with no bulging of the cheeks.)
- **Time:** 3 to 11 minutes.
- **To End:** Inhale deeply and then hold the breath for 10 to 15 seconds while you stretch the spine and tighten every fiber of your body. Cannon fire out the exhalation. Repeat this sequence two more times. Relax. Close your practice with one long "Sat Nam" (which loosely means *truth is my identity*) with your hands in prayer pose.

You can progress to doing full Kundalini Yoga sets, but start small and commit to daily practice first. My practice has included everything from 90 days of a Kundalini kriya to Wim Hof breathing and push-ups, to Qigong Awakening to Vitality series, to yoni egg exercises, the Five Tibetans movement, and binaural beats. The goal is to create a dedicated sacred time to go inward and send that ultimate signal of intention to grow beyond the trappings of your daytime reality.

## Travel Tips

### Tip #1: Use Flower Essences for Support

I have found energy medicine, specifically flower essences, to be a godsend during times of the Dark Night. Healer Joseph Aldo showed me how flower essences can support the clearing of old patterns and the integration of new beliefs, as well as alleviate symptoms quickly and efficiently. Unlike conventional medication, these remedies do not suppress what is arising; instead, they allow for understanding of the causes, supporting the full assimilation of the experience while minimizing pain and suffering.[14]

If you find yourself in the Dark Night, try using these specific flower essences for support.

- **Aspen** is beneficial when anxiety and fears of the unknown arise.

- **Cherry plum** supports those times when there is a fear of letting go, of losing control and having a mental/emotional breakdown.

- **Elm** is helpful for feelings of overwhelm due to stressors of inner transformation, when daily tasks and responsibilities are simply impossible to attend to.

- **Gorse** helps when feelings of depression and hopelessness are present.

- **Mimilus** quells everyday fears, such as the fear of death, failure, pain, poverty, or the future.

- **Mustard** clears temporary feelings of depression/melancholy, as if a dark cloud has descended out of nowhere and for no apparent reason.

- **Pine** is useful when there is guilt, self-criticism, or negative self-image.

- **Rescue remedy** is helpful for the initial stages of any traumatic experience to quickly reestablish equilibrium.

- **Star of Bethlehem** is a healing balm that neutralizes past shock and trauma, thereby restoring the self-healing mechanism of the body/mind.

- **Sweet chestnut** is the foremost remedy for the Dark Night of the Soul, as it addresses feelings of extreme despair, dejection, and loneliness. It is to be taken when one has reached "rock bottom" where there are helplessness, isolation, and the feeling of being utterly lost inside.

- **Walnut** is the "breaker of spells" and assists in cutting cords with the past. It helps in making healthy transitions when stuck in old paradigms or caught in relationships that no longer serve.

### Tip #2: Tap to Release Tension

EFT, Emotional Freedom Techniques, can be a line of

support in crisis and also an everyday self-healing tool. Also called *tapping*, this self-directed methodology reprograms your thoughts through acupressure point stimulation and affirmations, and allows the body to let go of traumatic life experiences by calming the nervous system and sending the body a signal of safety.[15]

**Tip #3: Create a Ritual for Medication Closure**

The following ritual, consisting of a simple exercise and a chant, was created jointly by me and my online VMR participants.

When you encounter your final prescription of medication, consider writing beliefs about yourself, your body, and your mind that led you to take the prescription in the first place. Write them on little strips of paper and put them in the empty prescription bottle. These can include:

- I am broken.
- I am sick.
- I was born with problems.
- My symptoms scare me and worry others.
- My chemistry is off.
- My body is so out of whack that I need meds to feel okay.
- Why should I suffer when I can just take medication?

Keep this bottle in a small box and refer to it if you are feeling scared or having a crisis of faith. Know that these beliefs were a reflection of your pain that you are now courageous enough to heal. It can help to recite the following chant aloud or silently to yourself:

# Ode to the Final Dose

*Today is my Independence Day.*

*It is the day that I pause, I breathe, and I turn back to see the many steps I have taken in my journey to this moment.*

*A journey that started with deep hurting. With feelings of abandonment, inadequacy, and betrayal. Feelings that I was not taught how to be with. Feelings that only grew louder and more chaotic the more I tried to suppress them.*

*Feelings that scared me so that I grew numb, heavy, and disconnected. I lost faith and felt life as an experience of crushing overwhelm and wrongness.*

*I felt broken and bad.*

*So, when I was told I was broken, when I was told that there was a way to fix this mess inside me, I naturally took the prescription. I took the label. And I wanted to believe it would help.*

*But there was always a small whisper that said, This is not the way. There's another way, and you will find it . . .*

*Today, I honor that whisper. Because that whisper is becoming my song. The song that I am here to sing. That only I can sing to the world.*

*I thank this medication for showing me who I am not, so I can understand who I am.*

*I understand that the betrayal I feel about a system and doctors who kept me sick and uninformed is simply the feeling of an illusion crumbling.*

*I see now that I needed every single moment of my journey, as hard as it has been, in order to arrive here, consecrating my rebirth, coming home to my true self.*

*A self that is ready to protect my inner child, to honor this child's experience with compassion, and to develop a deep intimacy with all of the feelings that need conscious expression and attention.*

*I am becoming that strong, clear, and calm adult who smiles a Buddha smile at the mystery of it all and who can witness— who is witnessing—the energies swirling around but who is not swept up by them, chaotically, desperately, or fearfully.*

*Today I commit to curiosity as my first response to triggering of fear, anger, or shame. I commit to always learning more about myself in service of the healing I deserve and the healing of my community and this planet. If I misstep, if my faith falters, it will only deepen my empathic connection to those who are still struggling, lost, and disempowered.*

*I am ready. I am chosen for this path. I will transform my pain into power with fierce compassion. May this final pill move through my system and take with it all of the myths, lies, illusions, and old ways of being, thinking, and behaving. For this chapter is closed, the tethers of disempowerment severed.*

*I am my own doctor, and I dedicate myself to myself. I commit to go inward and to ask questions and learn the dialect of my body. It will take time, and I trust that this wisdom will come to me more and more as I experience unconditional love for myself and the gift of simply being.*

C３ ８Ｏ

## What's Next . . .

After an experience of your body's power to heal, you will free up energy that can then be put toward reorganizing and reexamining elements of your life that are keeping you stuck—your beliefs, your relationships, your career or job, your orientation toward conventional medicine, and your access to living life with faith in a grand design of purpose and flow.

In Part III, Get Free, we will explore how to move forward in these areas now that you've broadened your horizons through expanded information and opened to a deeper connection with yourself. We start with adjusting your lens of perception—the bedrock foundation for any truly effective change—in Chapter 8.

# PART III

# GET FREE

Chapter 8

# THE LENS
# OF YOUR
# PERCEPTION

*Understanding is a handmaiden which can only wait
upon, or clarify, that knowledge, deeply born.*

— AUDRE LORDE

In this chapter, we look at the single most important thing you can do to start living in a way that integrates your new truth: to shine a bright light on every aspect of your life that is still reflecting an old fear-based pattern. Only then can you consciously choose to live, instead, from your newfound empowerment. I'll show you why and how to take inventory of your old beliefs in this chapter, and then in the remaining chapters, I'll show you how to integrate your new beliefs and reclaim important areas of your life.

## THE NEED FOR A WIDER LENS

As you move through the process of reclaiming your authentic self, or coming home to yourself, at some point you have to confront the ultimate layer of illusion. This is the perception that your life, this world as you see it, "just happens." That bad things and mistakes are truly what they seem, and you have no control over them.

But you do. For your day-to-day experience of life to feel more easeful, you have to zoom out and adjust your view of things. When you widen the lens of your perception, you see that there are no bad things and mistakes, but rather that everything happening is actually a reflection of your subconscious beliefs and conditioned behaviors. And it may be happening in service of *demonstrating* that to you. You begin to see that you are part of something more grand, the design of which becomes perceptible when your consciousness is ready to see it. How to live in that awakened state of reality is the subject of Chapter 10, but here I want to support you in making that shift, that adjustment to your lens of perception, so you can develop an inner compass for making choices to lead you there.

The state of *wonder* characterizes the awakened state; if we were all really awake, we'd be weeping tears of awe upon simply opening our eyes in the morning. But more typically, we think of life as a test to get an A on, a perspective that precludes any sense of wonder, keeping us on the hamster wheel of survival mode.

Survival perspective keeps you struggling and stressed. It's in our culture: Have you noticed that we are conditioned, as a society, to fight? We are at war with our symptoms (Beat cancer! Beat depression!) using anti-hypertensives, antidepressants, and antibiotics. We are at war with the bad guys (terrorists, criminals, Republicans/ Democrats). We are at war with nature (germs, weeds, green space).

And it's because we feel disconnected and disjointed. We aren't tapped into what many refer to as the quantum field, so we see everything from the atomized perspective of pieces and parts—not the whole.

## IMPORTANCE OF MINDSET

Today, mindset has become the bedrock of my transformational medicine practice and my activist mission, which is to awaken as many people as possible to their inbuilt healing capacity. My patients are invited to explore, examine, and become deeply aware of their beliefs. These beliefs determine how they experience suffering and the potential for self-healing activation. These beliefs give them the ability to trust that everything is going to be exactly as it needs to be.

If you are ready, it should be clear to you now that there is deep meaning in any illness, and that there is a corresponding invitation in that illness, one that is designed especially for you. In this way, how you interpret your symptoms—your perception of them—is everything.

Consider how your perceptions can make you sick in regard to the experience of stress. It's common knowledge that chronic, unmanaged stress can make you sick, while good stress, or *eustress*, helps you grow. So it's not the stress per se that makes you sick, but the *perception* of the stress that determines whether you send your body a signal of danger or safety.

In a recent review researchers refer to this definition of stress as a sensed threat to the body's state of stability, in which the response depends on, among other things, an organism's perception of the stressor and the perceived ability to cope with it.[1] McEwen has written about the role of perception in the stress response that leads to bodily expression of illness.[2] He refers to the burden on your body-mind as *allostatic load*, with perception of stress playing a major part in the development of physiologic response and illness.

Another report showed that the response to a simple question was the most meaningful determinant in whether or not a person would get a cold: *In general, how would you rate your health?*[3] After being inoculated with cold viruses, participants in Cohen's study demonstrated that negative health perception led to the *experience* of common cold symptoms regardless of whether the immune system was reacting. In other words, if someone had a positive health perception, got exposed, and had antibody confirmation of immune response, they did not manifest clinical symptoms of the cold (aka get sick).

## MAKE THE SHIFT

My patient Tasha wanted to be free from obsessive ruminations and the Zoloft she'd been taking for eight years for this so-called obsessive-compulsive disorder. Her mind often got stuck in a mode that had her irrationally thinking she was going to face a cancer diagnosis, contract an STD, or get a deadly infection. To say these worries took up a lot of real estate in her mind is an understatement. She also felt exhausted, constipated, cloudy, and emotionally flat on a day-to-day basis.

Tasha's obsessions were a reflection of her deeply held beliefs. They were landing on fertile soil and sprouting abundant weeds, making her believe:

- I can't trust my body.
- I feel completely out of control.
- Bad luck is random and imposed upon hapless victims.
- A diagnosis is a fate.
- If only I prepare and act fastidiously enough, everything will feel good.

If, like Tasha, such "weeds" characterize your belief system, you too are probably stuck in a loop of worrying that leaves you exhausted and emotionally drained. But it is your beliefs, not your circumstances, that are responsible for your state of mind. Your mind has served you well. It has kept you ahead of the game. It has helped you prepare. It has solved problems. Your mind only responds, however, to your felt beliefs, some of which don't serve you but have lured you into dark and airless places, holding you hostage in disconnection from your true self. Your mind will continue to try to provoke you, but it will obey and submit if you radiate a truth stronger than its claims and statements.

With a shift in your perception, you can embrace new beliefs to create a new mindset that is aligned with the result of your experience of bodily healing (the one-month protocol) to reflect new truths, like:

- My body is resilient in sophisticated ways.
- I have a capacity to heal if I support myself holistically.
- There is deep meaning to my symptoms and to the challenges I face.
- I trust that I will move through any and all difficulties that come my way—that I have what it takes.
- There is so much more to the story of human health and disease than we have been told by media, doctors, and drug companies.

If *these* are your truths, worry and obsessive anxieties and ruminations will necessarily wither. You'll be able to look at your thoughts more impartially, even with curiosity. In that inquiry, you may find, in fact, that there are hurt places, deep sadness, and raw loneliness beneath your anxious worries. But with a shifted belief system, you are able to go into those shadows and sit with them and grieve. You see how your obsessions and compulsions spring from conditioned fears about the world and your lack of control in this dangerous place called life, and you accept that. You see the purpose in it, that it was not random. Through this process of acceptance, you are able to bring forth a clear, focused mind and emotions, a healthy body, and a thriving soul.

## WIRED FOR BELIEF

You've seen the scientific validation for the power of your beliefs (placebo and nocebo) in Part I, but many still dismiss the placebo effect's having a positive impact on outcomes. This is due to the assumption that chemical drugs work through their specific "mechanism of action." But we now have provocative results of a new, well-designed study showing that what you believe, your mindset, is the most powerful predictor of clinical outcomes in psychiatry.[4]

In this randomized clinical trial, people with social anxiety disorder were divided into two groups, "overt" and "covert." Everyone was given 20 mg of a commonly prescribed SSRI, Lexapro, for nine weeks. In the overt group, people were told that they were being prescribed Lexapro, but in the covert group, people were told that they were given an "active placebo" that had similar side effects as the SSRI but had no clinical effects—even though they were given the same dosage of Lexapro as the overt group.

Their progress was monitored by fMRI scans, a type of brain imaging that measures the activity of brain regions. Even though both groups received the same SSRI dosages, 50 percent of people in the group told they were given Lexapro responded to treatment, while the response rate in the group told they were given placebo was a mere 14 percent. In fact, people in both groups had the same amount of Lexapro and its metabolites in their bodies. The only difference in their treatment was what they were told. Nearly four times as many people showed clinically significant improvement when they were told that they were receiving an SSRI instead of an active placebo. People in the overt group enjoyed reduced anxiety scores over the course of the study compared to people receiving the same SSRI dosage but told they were receiving a placebo.

Brain scans showed different neurological responses between the overt and covert groups. Generally speaking, people in the overt group showed increased neuronal reactivity in brain regions that are associated with cognition, attention, and rumination.[5]

Perhaps the knowledge that they were receiving an SSRI kicked off a cascade of thoughts about getting better. Further, the amygdala, the brain region associated with fear-based, fight-or-flight responses, showed different effects in terms of activation and connectivity based on the information given about treatments.[6] For example, people in the covert group exhibited increased activation of the amygdala and connectivity between the amygdala and the posterior cingulate cortex, which tracked with higher levels of anxiety.

This study shows we are wired for belief, so perhaps the most empowering thing we can do is to simply examine, expose, and understand what it is that we *actually* believe. To know this is to lay the tracks that your human experience and potential for healing will naturally follow. Shift your mindset to encompass what's possible, and the formerly impossible will become real for you.

## YOUR MIND CAN SHAPE REALITY

If you still need convincing about the powerful reality-shaping tool that your mind represents, consider the following scenario.

It's nighttime and you are walking down a dark alley alone. You hear footsteps rapidly approaching from behind. What's going to happen? Your mouth goes dry, your heart starts pounding, your breath quickens, and images of impending catastrophe arise in your mind. But then you suddenly hear a familiar voice over the sound of those footsteps. That entire cascade of fear reverses, and you may even start laughing to release the tension. The only thing that changed, of course, was your perception that there was danger. Your mind commandeered your body.

What if we *fully* embraced belief in the body's radical ability to heal? Cases often referred to as a spontaneous remission abound, but are considered anomalies. Perhaps when intention, thoughts, and emotions are aligned for growth, change, and self-discovery, spontaneous healing of the body *is* the predictable outcome.

We know the body can heal itself, but we have been interfering with it for so many decades—with Tylenol, antibiotics, steroids, and the like—that we have shifted expectations for just how rapidly and completely it can do so. But what if we were raised in a culture that believed more in the vital power of the body to heal, even spontaneously, rather than in one that believes we need man-made chemicals to outsmart it?

A contemporary example of such healing was demonstrated in a Harvard study.[7] Twelve patients with fractures were randomized to treatment with follow-up x-ray studies over 12 weeks. One group was guided in healing hypnosis and the other wasn't. The hypnotized group healed 2.5 weeks faster than the non-hypnotized group.

Power of the mind? Seems so.

## QUANTUM BIOLOGY: SEE YOURSELF WELL

Another way to explain the power of belief to shape physical outcomes—and engage you in seeing through a different lens—calls on quantum mechanics and something called the *observer effect.* It turns out that the observation of something can actually affect the thing being observed, stemming from the understanding that quantum physics has displaced the notion of an objective, measurable reality.

Here's how I apply this observer effect from quantum physics when I meet with patients: simultaneous to our interactions and co-presence, I am deeply engaged in visualizing them *well*. I see them in my mind's eye and feel them in my heart as the well version of themselves: their energy, appearance, voice, and the kind of wonder and awe that invariably accompany awakening to robust and resilient health. Seeing past the overt content of an interaction and connecting to the vital essence of that person, I bypass all of the stories, the blocks, and the interference between them and their potential for transcendence. I do this for my patients, but you can do this for others, and you can do this for *yourself*.

Quantum informational biology is beginning to explain how and why this experiential envisioning has its impact. One theory is that of *morphic resonance,* a phenomenon described by the brilliant renegade scientist and theorist Rupert Sheldrake in his book *A New Science of Life* and discussed in greater detail in *The Presence of the Past.*[8]

Sheldrake proposes that self-organizing systems draw on a collective memory to determine their path forward. A fetus grows into a baby simply because it has happened before, and thus the growth process can draw from what Sheldrake calls *morphogenetic fields.* Such fields contain a template for new experiences to conform to, based on an outcome that has already existed. This means that when one person heals from a previously incurable illness, it makes it easier for others to heal in the future, and this is the reason I have dedicated myself to supporting more and more seemingly "impossible" forms of healing.

Dr. Joe Dispenza, in his incredible books *Breaking the Habit of Being Yourself, You Are the Placebo,* and *Becoming Supernatural,* takes the process of healing one step further, teaching meditation techniques that involve the felt experience of an exalted emotion (love, gratitude, compassion) after accessing the subconscious through an open-focus meditation that frees the participant from ideas of self, time, and body. He has researched the ways in which optimizing energy fields through this intention to move beyond programmed thought connects us to the body's innate healing capacity, and to the unified field of infinite possibilities. The results can defy any understanding we have of the way disease is supposed to progress and disable, with near spontaneous reversals of chronic illness—no doctor's visit required.

## MEDICINE AS A BELIEF SYSTEM: SCIENTIFIC DOGMA

Shifting your mindset requires looking not only at your personal beliefs, but at the larger belief system that holds together our scientific worldview.

Rupert Sheldrake has this to say on the matter in *The Science Delusion*: "We are, many of us, waking up from a several century long slumber induced by Scientism—the dogmatic belief in the dominant narrative of science as religion. As we wake up . . . to new science that defies the old . . . Scientism believers will become more and more uncomfortable. . . . They may foam at the mouth and threaten violence at the suggestion that Scientism's sacred cows (pharmaceuticals, bioengineered foods, industrial chemicals) are not what we have been led to believe. Stay strong and reconnect to the elegance of a world of natural design, harmony, and regeneration."[9]

In his book, Sheldrake showcases 10 dogmatic beliefs that contemporary science believers have adopted from 400 years of entrenched and unexamined ideology. He describes these believers as materialists: those who believe that only matter is real, and in the purposeless, soul-less survival of the fittest. It's Sheldrake's assertion that science is stymied because of the questions we are not allowed to ask when we hold these assumptions as concrete and unchangeable laws.

Here are dogmas he feels should be reexamined:

- *Nature is mechanical*—Life is genetically programmed.
- *Matter is unconscious*—Inanimate objects cannot have consciousness.

- *The laws of nature are fixed*—They have not changed since the Big Bang.

- *Conservation of matter and energy*—The total amount is the same, forever.

- *Nature is purposeless*—There is no overarching design in nature and no higher purpose.

- *Heredity is solely biological*—Traits are passed down through genes alone.

- *The mind is inside the head and brain*—Thoughts cannot influence the outside world.

When we bring everything into question, we can dispassionately appreciate where our desire for comfort and security ends and where an independent search for truth begins. To pursue this truth, we must acknowledge where and how science has become a religion, and how medicine has become a matter of belief, with a zero-tolerance policy for critical inquiry.

Dr. Gonzalez wrote to me in a personal e-mail, "The last remaining religion is medicine. If you look at Sloan Kettering, it's actually like a temple, and the priests wear white coats and they speak their own language. Patients tend to bow down to that. Never underestimate the power of authority."

What happens when medicine masquerades as religion and seeks to summarily eliminate all competing belief systems? When we are told there is one truth and that truth is consensus-driven medicine? Perhaps the legislation introduced across this country to eliminate religious and personal belief exemptions to vaccination are a symptom of this insidious process.

Dr. Gonzalez also wrote, "Patients have to do the treatment they believe in. Fear is an infectious disease. You can catch fear but you can't catch faith. That has to come from within." I have always practiced in this ethos. I know that fear can act like a nocebo, creating negative outcomes, but where there is faith in the body's ability to heal when properly supported, magical things can happen.

## EPIGENETICS AND THE TELEOLOGIC PERSPECTIVE

One of the most persistent beliefs that needs to shift is that of a genetically predetermined future of your health. It just isn't so.

Have you ever worried about getting breast cancer because your mom and aunt both had it? What about bipolar disorder or lupus? It may have felt like you have a ticking time bomb inside you, and you just want to know when it's going to go off.

But the old saw "It runs in my family" no longer means what we once believed it to.

When I was in training, I had one hour of nutrition education that essentially positioned food as caloric currency. Why would it matter if we were born with the diseases we would ultimately struggle with? In gene-based science, toxicant exposure, rest, nutrition, and relationships are clearly window-dressing considerations.

With the completion of the human genome project, however, we learned that we have fewer protein-coding genes than an earthworm. This means that the genes we thought made us who we are, didn't. We had to go back to the drawing board. Where on earth does our seemingly infinite uniqueness come from? How are diseases manifesting if not genetically?

These questions and discoveries led to the birth of a new science and a new "teleologic" perspective, focusing on the purposes rather than causes of a phenomenon. It is named *epigenetics*. Epigenetics encompasses all that is beyond the genes (it actually means "above") and includes modulators, modifiers, and any influence on the expression of genes, and even the possibility that nonhuman genes may play an expressive role in human physiology. It also refers to the almost 99 percent of our genome that was once pejoratively called "junk DNA" and now is more mystically referred to as "dark matter," as Dr. Jeff Bland describe it at a 2016 Functional Forum event.[10]

One of the most powerful examples of the relevance of epigenetics is the lore of the "breast cancer gene." Angelina Jolie and many other women, even those in so-called natural health arenas, have succumbed to the hex or the belief that they are cursed by their genes, doomed to develop diseased breasts, ovaries, and uteruses if they just go on living with them in their bodies.

The literature itself claims that gene mutations such as the "breast cancer gene," or BRCA, seem to be doing different things *over time.* Doesn't that mean, by definition, that we are talking about *epigenetics?* Because the risk of a gene itself should not change over time. An oft-cited study concludes: "Risks appear to be increasing with time: Breast cancer risk by age 50 among mutation carriers born before 1940 was 24%, but among those born after 1940 it was 67%."[11]

In a timely meta-analysis entitled "Worse Breast Cancer Prognosis of BRCA1/BRCA2 Mutation Carriers: What's the Evidence?" the authors conclude: "Our review shows that, in contrast to currently held beliefs of many oncologists and despite 66 published studies, it is not yet possible to draw evidence-based conclusions about the association between BRCA1 and/or BRCA2 mutation carriership and breast cancer prognosis."[12]

This reflects a more modern understanding that only about 1 percent of diseases are truly genetic in nature (i.e., due to a congenitally inherited and irreversible gene defect), and that we may very well have misunderstood our interpretation of these genes' functions. The rest is lifestyle. In other words, we create our experience and determine our destiny: *epigenetics.*

As we embrace our agency in our own bodily experience, we must embrace complexity and take off the blinders of our one gene, one ill, one pill model of thinking. As you open your mind to this shift underfoot—a shift into a more ecological type of medicine, a more collaborative, communal, and connected type of medicine—revel in what the more beautiful science is showing us about our need to let go of what we once believed. It served us, but its time has passed. Now it's time to recognize that it's not happening to us; it *is* us, asking to be healed.

*The fairest thing we can experience is the mysterious. It is the fundamental emotion which stands at the cradle of true art and true science . . . the mystery of the eternity of life, and the inkling of the marvelous structure of reality, together with the single-hearted endeavor to comprehend a portion, be it ever so tiny, of the reason that manifests itself in nature.*

— ALBERT EINSTEIN

## EMBRACE UNCERTAINTY: MAYBE MIND

So how can you shift your mindset from one of disempowering fear to one of empowered belief? It's not as hard as you might think. First you must make a conscious choice to trade in your old beliefs and cultivate some new ones. This is easier once you've had a felt experience of your body's power to heal by undergoing the one-month Reset protocol described in Chapter 6. You can then begin to reprogram your belief system by practicing a simple technique called *Maybe Mind.*

What is Maybe Mind? We have a natural tendency to love simplicity and certainty. But the reason for that is our mind's love of control. In order for the mind to feel comfortable, it needs to sense mastery over a given situation or circumstance—no wonder we are crawling out of our own skins! And when things are simple, they feel manageable and familiar, which makes us feel safe.

The truth is that it is a fear response we all engage in, and that "sitting in the gray" is a learned skill that we can all strive for.

A Chinese parable you may have heard demonstrates the value of developing the skill of Maybe Mind, so you can engage your curiosity and inquire as to the meaning of events:

Once upon a time, there was a Chinese farmer whose horse ran away. That evening, all of his neighbors came around to commiserate. They said, "We are so sorry to hear your horse has run away. This is most unfortunate."

The farmer said, "Maybe."

The next day the horse came back, bringing seven wild horses with it, and in the evening everybody came back and said, "Oh, isn't that lucky. What a great turn of events. You now have eight horses!"

The farmer again said, "Maybe."

The following day his son tried to break one of the horses, and while riding it, he was thrown and broke his leg. The neighbors then said, "Oh dear, that's too bad," and the farmer responded, "Maybe."

The next day the conscription officers came around to conscript people into the army, and they rejected his son because he had a broken leg. Again all the neighbors came around and said, "Isn't that great!"

Again, he said, "Maybe."[13]

The Chinese farmer experiences fortune and tragedy equally as "maybe good, maybe bad," with every occurrence holding potential energy for an unexpected consequence or benefit. The message here is to see that there may be a design too complex to perceive from your vantage point, to appreciate that nothing is simple or certain and that there are multiple narratives underpinning each and every happening—even when those happenings are dark and disturbing.

Nature is an integrated process of immense complexity, and it is impossible to tell whether anything that happens in it is good or bad. You never know what will be the consequences of the misfortune or good fortune, so you're best to adopt an attitude of "sitting in the gray" and embracing uncertainty.

## The Victim and the Anthropologist

**Play a game:** When the shroud of blackness descends upon your worldview, it's time to play a game that will open you up to seeing through different lenses of perception. In my workshops, I call this game "The Victim and the Anthropologist." Here are the steps I ask my participants to take:

1. Focus on a challenging past experience.

2. Narrate this experience, in your mind, on paper, or to someone else, *through the lens of the victim*—i.e., the person who has bad luck, has been the target of lots of horrible things, and is fundamentally helpless to change any aspect of this hopeless life.

3. Tell the same story, but now *through the lens of the anthropologist.* What would someone see who is dispassionately assessing the situation? Can you inhabit another perspective? Can you become curious and imagine that perhaps it's not, in fact, all about you, and that people make decisions all the time for myriad reasons?

4. Get even more curious and inquire: Perhaps you co-created a dynamic—meaning it takes two to tango—and you invited this kind of energy, attention, or treatment in some way. How can you own your part, even if it is a belief about danger, oppression, or unfairness that was then reflected back to you in real-life circumstances.

Here's an example: Your house burned down. Is this instance a horrific, senseless nightmare that confirms your unlucky lot in life? Or is that the reason you stayed with your Aunt Sally whose friend's son Rob stopped by to drop off a package . . . and now you and Rob are madly in love and talking about starting a family!

## KATIE'S STORY: COMING HOME TO HERSELF

At age 19, Katie was diagnosed by her family doctor with anxiety and obsessive-compulsive disorder. Thus began a decade of what she referred to as "managing my mental disorder" with a myriad of prescription drugs: Effexor to Prozac to Vyvanse to Lexapro to Zoloft. "And on top of those, always Xanax as needed," she commented. But not one of those drugs ever "fixed" her.

During those years, Katie searched endlessly for the "real fix"—that one thing that would finally get her anxiety and OCD under control. She tells of her ordeal: "One counselor spent our entire first session reading me descriptions of my diagnoses from her *DSM* book.

I felt like I was sinking as she read on and on, describing generalized anxiety, social anxiety, depression, and OCD. I felt devastated as she concluded with 'Yup, that fits you!' and then said, 'These are things you will always have, but we will work together on strategies to help you cope.' I felt sick. I left and never went back. Today I realize that the sick feeling was not because of the bleak prognosis she gave me, but because I knew that she was wrong."

It was not out of stubbornness or denial that Katie refused to believe her doctor that day. It was something inside her that knew the truth: a truth that despite years of being dismissed, she refused to give up. "I had no idea what that truth was or even looked like, but my body and mind knew it deep down. And they gently hung on until I was able to see it," she told me.

It was seeds of truth that began Katie's transformation, starting with her hearing my podcast interview about the drugs she had used and was still using, and about her diagnoses. Upon listening, she reported: "In a matter of minutes, everything I was told and believed about these topics began to fall apart. I was confused and angry. I sat in my car and cried because I felt so deceived. And because her words screamed hope."

She continues: "The main thing I learned from Dr. Brogan is that the most important key to my healing is my mind and my beliefs. When she told me a pill wasn't going to fix me and that I'm not broken, I shattered in relief. I shattered because they had never fixed me, and deep down I knew they never would. Everyone told me I had a disorder, a disease. She was the first and only person to tell me otherwise."

From that day forward, Katie proceeded with the understanding that her body is complex and that it wants to heal. She listened to her body and started giving it what it needed to function well, and when the body is functioning well, the mind changes. A whole new you emerges.

Her words are testimony to this: "The biggest change, however, is my mind. I feel calm. My racing thoughts no longer haunt me. The feeling of panic that drove me most days is no longer here. The impatience, irritability, and harshness I reacted with daily simply don't happen. I feel in control of my thoughts. I am present, happy, hopeful, and optimistic about life. I enjoy everyday things and no longer live in fear, dread, and overwhelm."

Katie recently weaned completely off Zoloft and experienced no return of symptoms while tapering. Instead, she felt more clear and present with every day that passed. Before, her anxiety was as much a part of her as her name; it defined her, and it defined her future. "I haven't spoken of 'my anxiety' in months now," she told me. "That is no longer me. I feel like I have returned, but 'I' is a me that I've never actually met until now."

Hearing Katie's story, you may think it hard and overwhelming to make so many changes, but according to her, "The only hard part is starting. Your mind knows the way, and once you help it along, the journey is easy—and you will feel free."

## Travel Tips

### Tip #1: The 17 Seconds Rule

The idea behind the 17 Seconds Rule is that if you can think a thought for at least 17 seconds, that thought will attract another thought of similar vibration.

This technique also makes it easier to shift your thoughts when you are in a negative head space. Once your thoughts are more positive, your emotions follow suit and your overall vibration starts lifting. It takes practice, but once you get the hang of it, the 17 Seconds technique can help you shift your mindset from one that is blocking you from receiving what you want to one that is open to it.

This is a powerful practice because it specifies a certain amount of time for you to focus on your positive thought. You can use the 17 Seconds Rule mentally, by speaking aloud to yourself or to someone else, or by writing it down. The important point, and what makes it work, is not to contradict your thought during that 17-second period.

The way I use the 17 Seconds Rule is this: Any time something exciting happens, I close my eyes for 17 seconds and set off emotional fireworks to program my attention around the fact that the event actually happened before moving on to the next thing that hasn't yet happened. And I also try to say thank you when someone compliments me (**instead of** *Oh, this? I got it on the sale rack at Rainbow!*).

**Tip #2: See Yourself Well**

Use the principle of morphic resonance from quantum mechanics to visualize and then manifest your further healing.

**Try it:** Meditate on wellness, on what it would feel like to be finally free and at ease in yourself, your mind, your heart. Ask yourself:

- What would my body look like? My skin, hair, eyes, muscle tone?

- What would my mind say to me in this well state?

- What would my heart feel: Peace? Joy? Love?

- Where is the energy most intense in my body when I am well? Is it rising up and out? Localized somewhere?

- What does the energy around me feel like? Light? Safe? Clear?

Feel all of this now as though it has happened, and you are already there in the experience of your wellness.

**Tip #3: Meditation for Connecting to Your Intuition**

For help in getting in touch with your deeper beliefs and intuition, try this Kundalini breathing exercise, called Two-Stroke Breath to Connect the Subconscious and the Intuition. Description:

- **Posture:** Sit cross-legged with a straight spine. Bend your arms at the elbows so your fingertips point upward. Place the hands, forearms, and elbows so they all make one vertical line from elbow to fingertips. Keep them in line with your chest. Rest your upper arms against your side ribs. Place your hands in gyan mudra (connect the thumb with the forefinger, tip to tip, with the other fingers relaxed) with the palms facing forward. Sit very straight with fingers straight and with a precise touch. The forearms must be perpendicular to the floor and in line with the body.

- **Eyes:** Eyes are nine-tenths closed and one-tenth open.
- **Breath:** Breathe in the following way (Trinity Breath): Slightly pucker your lips and inhale powerfully in two strokes through the mouth (1 second per stroke = 2-second inhalation). Exhale powerfully in one stroke through the nose (1 second).

**Time:** Continue for 15 minutes.

**To Finish:** Inhale deeply and put your hands together at the center of the chest in Prayer Mudra with the forearms parallel to the ground. Hold your breath for 15 to 20 seconds as you press your hands together with all your strength. Press so powerfully that your hands shake. Exhale. Inhale, hold the breath for 15 to 20 seconds and repeat this pressure on the hands. Exhale. Then inhale and stretch your arms up over your head and stretch your spine strongly upward. Hold the breath 15 to 20 seconds. Exhale and relax.[14]

CR BO

# What's Next . . .

In Chapter 9, we'll explore what it's like for you to come home to yourself as you take inventory of the important relationships in your life and how you live in community. It may be necessary to align the new you with a new social reality. Your job/career, as well as new attitudes about your habitual response to medical treatment, may also need to be aligned. I'll show you how you can do all this and create support for the everyday realities of your new life.

Chapter 9

# COMING HOME
# TO YOU

*You never change things by fighting the existing reality.*
*To change something, build a new model that*
*makes the existing model obsolete.*

— R. Buckminster Fuller

When you get clear on what your felt belief system consists of—
your *real* truth—it's time to run everything you do, say, and dedicate
yourself to through the lens of your new beliefs. This is the work
that is before you now: to make an assessment of important areas of
your life and decide what passes the test of authenticity and what
does not. If something doesn't, it will not withstand the bright light
of you-ness that is now shining. Time to upgrade! And it isn't about
a one-time house cleaning, but rather about an ongoing lifestyle of
integrity, lived one moment at a time.

In this chapter, we will explore the most important areas for
reassessment and integration: family relationships, marriage and
romantic relationships, community support, habitual response to
illness and the medical system, and choice of vocation/profession.
As we explore each of these pain points, I will offer guidance in
learning to navigate your new reality.

## FAMILY: COMING INTO HARMONY

It's said that if you think you are enlightened, try spending two weeks with your family. In your travels through your new life, family can represent the heaviest baggage of all, rife with shame, abandonment, and violation.

As you become someone different from who you were, your family may very well not like it. The eye roll your new diet gets from your mother, or the excommunication by your brother because of your unvaccinated baby. Beyond being a hall of mirrors for past experiences, family members—parents, siblings, and extended members—challenge you to *integrate*. If you remain in touch with them, you have to accept not only who *they* are as blood relatives, but also who *you* are when you are around them.

I believe that our families are here to teach us existential lessons about healing: healing from wounds of inadequacy and conditional self-love that family members themselves may have inflicted in our early childhoods. Presenting your newly birthed adult consciousness to your family members is an act of self-love and protection of your childself that will ultimately confer a deep sense of safety. It's time to stop playing the part you did, in service of an illusion of who you thought you were.

> *[T]o be ourselves causes us to be exiled by many others,*
> *and yet to comply with what others want causes us to*
> *be exiled from ourselves. It is a tormenting tension*
> *and it must be borne, but the choice is clear.*
>
> — Clarissa Pinkola Estés, Women Who Run with the Wolves

Women, in particular, are expert at meeting the imagined needs of others before identifying their own. Sounds lovely, but it leads to highly toxic dynamics because we don't know how to set appropriate boundaries (say no when we mean no) and we don't know what we feel, so we are always secretly hoping that someone will read our minds and meet our needs that we never even knew were there. In fact, my friend Dr. Christiane Northrup, who has been committed to healing and liberating women her entire career, most recently wrote a book called *Dodging Energy Vampires* describing what she feels is one of the top reasons empaths (highly sensitive people) get sick: toxic relationships.

As you begin to set healthy boundaries with family and represent who you really are, this will likely kick up some serious anxiety. You'll fear retaliation, judgment, or disappointment. Sit with that fear, knowing that it is old. Get to know it and recognize its signature essence so you can use your adult consciousness to say to your childself, *I see you, and am here to protect you.* As you work toward a more authentic dynamic with family members, you will feel pride in yourself . . . that's your childself's way of saying thank you.

One thing that might become clear before you flee your family and tell them all to enjoy their un-awakened lives is this: you are giving them your energy if you still feel triggered by them. Make peace, and in doing so, cut energetic cords—*before* cutting relationship cords.

Eastern philosophy tells us to find peace, satisfaction, and even joy in the mundanity of life. I believe there is deep truth here. Be okay with what is, first. When you aren't, and you focus all of your energy on what you want, or what you think should be, or what you desperately need to manifest, you lose an opportunity to neutralize the energetic pull of the circumstances you are looking to run from. And those circumstances—whether it's a relationship or a house or a job—will continue to pull on you through your fear, resistance, and negative emotion.

Owning your choices and beliefs, relinquishing the desire to convince anyone to join you, and knowing how to represent your needs as a calm, clear, self-possessed adult will begin to shift the energetics of your old family dynamics to make room for the new you.

---

*Our family are the people who know who you are, appreciate who you are, never want you to be anyone else, and love you regardless of where you end up or what false turns you take.*

— Dr. Nicholas Gonzalez

## Healing Your Childhood Wounds: Four Steps

- **Step #1: Journal your earliest memories.** First things first: Look under all of the stones in your childhood garden. Check out the creepy crawlies and see what's there. Write down the most disturbing recollections you have in your mind (it's okay to destroy what you've written afterward), express these memories to someone you trust, or just say them to yourself in the mirror. Put words to your experiences and beliefs so there isn't just this looming dark power over your consciousness.

  Take a minute to write down what you were told while growing up about money, sex, love, your body, disease, the environment/nature. What were all of the negative things ever said about you? These beliefs are in there, framing the stage of your life, choosing the characters, and directing the pit orchestra.

- **Step #2: Cultivate gratitude.** The best antidote for resentment is the feeling of gratitude. I remember my skepticism when I first read the data from HeartMath Institute about the potential of gratitude to bring the heart, lungs, and brain into electrical resonance or "coherence."[1] But it turns out that there's something powerful about this feeling. Try it. Focus on your heart, choose a soothing color, and imagine it misting out from your heart onto the elements of your life that you are most grateful for. The roof over your head, your two legs, your children's sticky hands, your iPhone. Just feel it.

  Try this meditation from Louise Hay, which involves recognizing the fact that we are all victims of victims: Envision your father, and then your mother, and then yourself as a frightened, crying toddler or child. Console this toddler version of each person and then shrink them down to a size that can fit into your heart.[2]

  As you place them there, you integrate and humanize those painful forces instead of resenting them. This doesn't let any parent off the hook for what might have been heinous behavior and unconscionable choices. It simply softens the hard places in you so you can heal.

- **Step #3: Release emotions through your body.** Anger and pain are real. They need to be felt, acknowledged, and released. Suppressing emotions steals your vital force energy. So reclaim that energy—you need it!

For releasing emotions, try Clarity Breathwork.[3] This is a powerful process of healing and transformation done in a chaperoned or group experience that involves generating states of release through hour-long breathing sessions. It deeply supports the clearing away of old energies, patterns, conditioning, negative thoughts, and emotions and opens the doors wide for new life and greater consciousness.

- **Step #4: Work with a family therapist.** I am also a huge believer in family therapy. For many of us, exploring deeper topics with family can feel like running naked onto a battlefield, and I will attest to its having been the most high-yield work I've done to honor my childself. Finding a therapist you can work with can help you find the courage to move through spaces you couldn't otherwise move through.

## WHEN VISITING WITH FAMILY

At holiday time and during visits home, you might find yourself hoping your family will finally see the real you. But instead of relying on hope, it's better to prepare yourself with these reminders:

- **Let strong emotions come up and pass through.** Don't attach a story to your emotions, allowing them to reinforce your held beliefs about your family. Remember they are here to help remind you that your wound is active, and that you are in a position to attend to it as a conscious adult. As feelings come up, consciously slow your breathing down so you can command your stress response.

- **Refrain from bringing up your medication taper journey if you are in the midst of that process.** Rather, wait to be asked about it. This is complex terrain for people to appreciate in both its physical and spiritual nature. Debating and arguing never work in this case. Just continue to commit to your self-care, over and over and over, and family members will eventually see the result.

- **Bless them.** Do this because your blessing may be the energetic tipping point in an otherwise stuck dynamic of old patterns. When you bless someone, you are large enough, abundant enough, and peaceful enough to do so. You allow another to be who they are, on their journey, in the best way they can. In blessing another, you release any expectation that they will finally save you, heal, or meet your needs in ways they never did and may never do.

- **Bring your own food and snacks.** Don't let the mob mentality of old patterns pull you off your path. Hold your space with conviction and strength, not preachiness or righteousness, which may require some grass-fed jerky in your bag.

- **Come home to your people.** After a visit, reconnect with those who you see as a touchstone after weathering challenging family interactions. Share your experience with them and then let it go.

## Travel Tip for Family Harmony: Cutting Cords Meditation

When I feel pulled into keeping score, blaming, or resentment, I stop, drop, and do a "cutting cords" meditation to free myself and restore boundaries. This meditation was recorded for me by one of my beloved teachers, Joseph Aldo, and is available on my website.[4]

When finding harmony with your family of origin is your priority, the path to honoring yourself while honoring others becomes apparent, and all you have to do is walk it. Whether you allow your experience of your family to passively unfold or you need to cut cords, you will *know* what to do (rather than reflexively react) when your body is healed and your mind is clear, so commit to self-care over and over again. Know that you will then be strong enough to navigate spaces you thought you would never touch with a 10-foot pole.

## ROMANTIC RELATIONSHIPS: HOW TO NAVIGATE

"I'm not sure I see us both walking down this path together . . . I think this is where we have to part ways. He sees how I've changed, but I don't think there's a cell in his body that is aware our partnership is functionally over."

Listening to Lucy that day, it occurred to me that I couldn't remember the last time a woman completed her tapering work with me and still had her primary romantic relationship—namely, marital partnership—intact. I calculated that I have an astronomical divorce rate from start to finish of the taper and transformation process.

I certainly don't advise or encourage my patients, most of whom have children, to end their marriages. But it can be a natural consequence that, in leaving behind the person you were, there are some relationships that remain at the headstone of that former self, perhaps arrested in a state of mourning or even denial. In the awakening process, it seems to be that the container of a marriage must, at times, be broken in order for this new empowered you to emerge.

Often, but not always. How will you know? Well, it depends on what you want.

Like Harville Hendrix and Helen LaKelly Hunt, David Deida, Kim Anami, Robert Augustus Masters, and others, I believe that the container of the romantic dyad can be a perfectly designed laboratory for two things: healing childhood wounds and experiencing the transcendent power of erotic energy to connect us to divinity. With the right kind of support, this primary relationship can offer you a sense of deep safety and sensual healing while also revealing your most primal wounds for the opportunity to heal.

Author and psychotherapist John Welwood describes relationship as a unique human opportunity for alchemical transformation, a chance to confront our latent fears of our own shadow energy. He writes: "Opening to another also flushes to the surface all kinds of conditioned patterns and obstacles . . . our deepest wounds, our grasping and desperation, our worst fears, our mistrust, our rawest emotional trigger points."[5]

In relationships, unresolved childhood wounds can perpetuate instability. In a fascinating study, researchers investigated the relationship between parenting style, inflammation, and later-life depression.[6] They concluded that early negative parenting elevates both inflammation and depressive symptoms during adulthood and increases the likelihood that problems in an adult relationship with a romantic partner will amplify inflammation still further, indirectly amplifying depressive symptoms.

*Romantic partnerships matter* because they can heal you or they can drive your soul to rebel in the form of so-called depressive episodes. In fact, the authors of the study reference another study showing that intimate partner relational problems were associated with a 2.7-fold increase in major depressive episodes in the following 12 months. These relationships can be a cage or a temple. This may be why, as my patients awaken to their essential selves, they need to break out of the marital construction they established while medicated . . . and the high divorce rate from start to finish of recovery work is proof that often these relationship dissolutions are part of a necessary shedding process.

So how can you heal your past in a present relationship? Maybe you suffered severe abuse—sexual, physical, or emotional. Or maybe your mother said something to you one day when you were seven that laid down the cellular programming for a fearful life. How do you integrate such dissonance and become whole again? Should you ignore it? Medicate it for the sake of your partner? Tough it out?

No. You want to get at the root of your beliefs and transform them with your compassionate awareness, because childhood trauma reverberates throughout adult relationships (platonic included). Here are some guidelines for healing childhood wounds as they come up in your romantic relationship, so you can thrive and grow:

## Healing in Relationships

**Know your triggers.** Ever have an extreme reaction to someone's behavior? Like your husband was eating crackers, and just the sound of his chewing made you want to strangle him? We all have different buttons that can get pushed, particularly when we are feeling stressed out, overwhelmed, or vulnerable. These "triggers" are set in place by your childhood experience, the sentinel traumas—micro or macro—to your nervous system, defining what danger looks like to you.

Note the pattern in when you get set off—agitated, hurt, affronted, defensive. When are you trying to be right about being wronged? Triggers are often marked by the feeling of "this isn't fair!"—the battle cry of the victim mindset, and the wounded child activating her defensive responses of control, manipulation, and the quest to be right. Becoming aware of these triggers is essential to recognizing the associated defenses and taking responsibility for your healing. Vulnerability can feel terrible, and it is the most direct route to exactly what we want—contact, connection, intimacy, and love.

**Maintain the vessel.** The crucible of a monogamous romantic relationship creates the commitment needed to sit in the shadow material that surfaces. There's nowhere to run, nowhere to source attention or intimacy, and no back-door conditional clauses. This is why and how a dyad of this nature can radically transform the energy of childhood wounding and shine a light on every and all shadowy blind spots so they too can be loved, and even made love to.

To maintain this powerful vessel, take inventory of the ways in which energy is being leaked. For many with a history of sexual abuse, flirtation and sexualized dynamics have become a means of feeling safe in the world, of feeling in control of otherwise unfamiliar power dynamics. Examine where you are flirting, where you are engaging the potential of past relationships, where you are leaving open the possibility of a sexualized energy outside the relationship. Also ask if you are leaking energy in your work, through boundaryless platonic relationships or other obsessive objects of attention. Put your relationship first and it will hold you through your transformation.

**Speak in feelings.** It can be irresistible to engage old defenses when you are triggered by a romantic partner. As you cultivate the capacity to observe this triggering, and your body becomes more and more of an informational vessel translating your heart energy (Is your chest tight? Your stomach in a knot? Your throat constricted?), you will develop the capacity to speak in terms of your triggers and feelings. You'll be able to say, *I suddenly feel anger rising up in my chest,* instead of *I hate when you do that!* Or even just *I'm triggered right now,* as an invitation to connect through basic touch or eye contact before engaging in any debates or high-level discussions. Feelings speak a very simple language. As someone who has mastered the art of hiding my childself and her vulnerability in a remote basement, I know the power of elaborate stories and narratives to obscure sentiments as simple as, "Do you love me?" If you have the courage (because this level of vulnerability can feel embarrassing and extremely uncomfortable) to show up with your childself in your heart and translate her simple toddler-level language, the ego swordfight may end right there.

## POLARITY IN RELATIONSHIPS

A critical aspect to the energetics of a healing romantic relationship is the concept of polarity or a complementary balance of power. In order for this balance to come about, *you have to choose whether you want to be the masculine or the feminine polarity.*

As Dr. Carl Jung taught, we all have an *anima* and *animus* within us, a female and male essence. It is an ever-present goal to nurture both sides, but one side is likely your dominant expression, independent of your gender, sexual orientation, or relationship predilections.

The sage and passionate David Deida, author of 10 books about the sexual and spiritual relationships between men and women, helps elucidate this essence in his prolific writings through a simple question: *Do you want to be ravished or do you want to ravish?* The feminine-essence person will have the deep desire to be ravished and to open in pleasure to her fullest expression of receptivity. We may have developed many reactive "shells," as he calls them, in striving toward acceptance and love: for example, a feminine shell of self-adornment, around a masculine shell of striving and career-devoted independence, around a tender feminine core that longs to be seen for her radiant energy.

Deida discusses the different stages of consciousness for the feminine and masculine. He sees feminine consciousness as growing from first-stage neediness, to second-stage independence (*I don't need a man* and *I can do anything he can do better*), to third-stage opening to the devotional yearning for the masculine complement through which to contact divinity. The feminine, according to Deida, wants fullness and love.

The masculine first stage is a focus on power and finance, the second stage a progression to making a service-oriented mark on the world, and the third stage a surrender to spiritual growth at all costs through a fearless commitment to resting in conscious presence around the light of the feminine. The masculine wants emptiness and freedom.

Together, these two forces, feminine and masculine, create the merger of consciousness and light and are themselves a technology for channeling the mystical energy of the quantum field.

Working within the concept of polarities helps us orient around the many layers of defenses and aspects of our habitual tendencies that are an extension of the wounding and papering over of our essence.

## THIS WOMAN'S WORK

Women, including myself and most of the women I know, have been swept up into several millennia of idolizing the masculine principles of doing, mastery, and control. Similarly, men have engaged this unbalanced masculine, living lives in which vulnerability, emotion, and deeper intuitive drives are considered weaknesses.

If you choose to cultivate your feminine principle, you cannot insist on controlling, planning, outsmarting, criticizing, and correcting your partner. That masculine energy will limit his emergence. And it will likely engender either a feminization of his energy or a duel of masculine poles. You may have to learn to take a deep breath and surrender even when you feel you know better, can do better, or are smarter. Not easy, but it's in service of softening and coming into a new kind of intuitive, receptive, and creative power that inspires action without directing. It's in service of relinquishing the healing-sabotaging need to be right. If this is the kind of growth you want to do for yourself as an individual, it may very well be that romantic relationship is the grounds for your own spiritual evolution.

I believe that what women (or the feminine polarity in the relationship) want is protection. You might assume that this would be protection from the forces of danger out in the world, but what we really want is the sacred masculine to rise up and help protect us from our own shadow. For example, when I feel vulnerable (i.e., feel I might be judged, abandoned, or unloved), I kick into high masculine gear and start to mentalize and intellectually make the case that I have a better/deeper/more accurate understanding about what is going on. My personal shadow hallmark is that I feel an urgency to communicate my perspective (aka control the narrative). This takes me out of my heart and out of connection, and keeps me from feeling the fear of abandonment, sense of inadequacy, or shame that is driving the defensive behavior. If my partner is not clear enough or present enough to help me see these blind spots, I may struggle to come to know them myself. I may forfeit the opportunity to learn how to respond non-reactively to my triggers so I can finally allow my childself feelings to be felt, acknowledged, and contained by my adult consciousness.

Most powerful women have not learned to work with our emotional energy (and sensitivity) consciously (because we were raised afraid to feel vulnerable), and we want to be guided by someone who loves us enough to contain us, call us out, and help hold us accountable to our highest expression and nothing less. So when we are employing our defenses and controlling habits, the masculine says, *Stop and feel what you're trying to defend against . . . I can help you experience, acknowledge, and honor this emotion instead of reacting to it.*

This is a kind of merger that results from boundaries (what do I need and how can *I* work to understand and even meet that need?) and an ever-expanding sense of personal responsibility for our experience. The less we judge, the less we expect, and the more curious we can become about the other's experience, the deeper the capacity for sacred contact through the relationship.

Becoming an adult and breaking free of patterns that leave us feeling half human involve expanded emotional capacity. Specifically, they involve a deepening okay-ness with incredibly intense feelings of fear, anger, shame, rejection, and abandonment. Instead of getting swept up into the old defensive structure that kept you from fully feeling or experiencing the present reality—eating, avoiding, withdrawing, or in my case mentalizing and artfully defending my perspective—you simply *choose* to feel. You have an internal acknowledgment that you are safe, that your childhood abuser is not before you, that your parents are not in the room, and that you are grown enough to handle the storm inside and let it simply exist. Being an adult means you are strong enough to choose to watch and open even though all your personality wants to do is wince and close. This is how we become adults rather than children wearing 100 layers of clothing and pretending to be big.

Romantic relationship can be an incredibly powerful technology for adultification, as well as a conduit for the organizing principal of divinity to emerge in little pockets around the globe. In fact, I believe that the cultivation of the sacred masculine and the divine feminine is what will save this planet, one healing relationship at a time. And that's because eros is the antidote to the rational materialism that tells us we are floating on a dead rock in the middle of nowhere subjected to random forces of danger and detriment. Emotion, sensuality, and pleasure emerge from a worldview that tells us we are here, having a human experience simply in order to be, feel, and know the power and mystery of what is.

## Travel Tips for Navigating Relationships

### Tip #1: Be Curious

When you are feeling wronged, affronted, or otherwise misunderstood, shift out of blame and into curiosity. Ask what's going on here, and commit to witnessing your partner's experience. Two truths can indeed exist simultaneously. Choosing to place love and trust in the foreground is likely to generate experiences that reflect the wisdom of this choice. Rather than assuming certainty, commit to exploring the possibility that your partner has something to show you that you can't quite see. In the end, what you're feeling is likely a long-neglected and very real emotion from your childhood or even your ancestry, so can you possibly feel gratitude for the opportunity this conflict is generating? It's an opportunity to feel what is already yours, within.

### Tip #2: Truth-Telling

Set aside one hour a week to look into each other's eyes and listen to a sharing that might otherwise have gone unsaid.

Share something you were afraid to express and commit to receiving whatever your partner chooses to share, with a focus on feelings rather than the details.

**Tip #3: Learn Your Partner's Triggers**

Often referred to as love languages, we each have different ways that we feel love. Know your partner's vulnerabilities related to his/her past trauma. Learn how to show them love in a way that may feel less than natural or even comfortable for you. Maybe he is triggered by a harsh tone of voice and she is triggered by unanswered communications. In a climate of personal responsibility and a commitment to self-love, having a partner meet these needs is spiritual gravy on top. Explore these patterns together so the ghosts of the past can gracefully exit the relationship.

## COMMUNITY: THE MAGIC OF THE TRIBE

As your new life unfolds, you will want to surround yourself with mirrors of your highest potential to curate the right (new) support network. After the initial work done during the one-month Reset program, you've liberated the energy you needed to finally get your relationships aligned. No one can go through profound transformation alone. We need each other to recover—and to thrive.

While I advocate for diet and nutrition as the portal to wellness, participants in VMR claim that community may be the most critical element of their healing journey. The online group is an incredibly powerful healing space, and I am inspired daily by the exchanges posted by participants. Others will find a community through conscious living: through a holistic group, your local yoga or meditation studio, your children's Waldorf school, or maybe even through tea with someone you strike up a conversation with at the bookstore.

However you may get support, when you awaken to your true self, your soul family hears that call, and they come. These new friendships, romantic dynamics, and collaborative partnerships emerge from the fabric of your new life experience. And you will know when you find these people because you will feel like you can be yourself with them. They will come into your sphere effortlessly, once you let them. They will reflect to you your highest potential and hold an image of you even when you feel lost and disconnected from it.

## Community Wounds

We are social animals, and our health and wellness depend on it. We used to wake up to dozens of eyes, but now in our modular homes and digitized worlds, we no longer feel that our tribe is holding us. More connected, and yet less fulfilled, our wired lives leave our social needs superficially met while the wound can fester below, a reality explored in the article "The Effect of Mobile Phone Use on Prosocial Behavior."[7]

Our unmet primal needs can manifest as addiction-like behaviors as we seek to medicate deficiencies like that of not having a tribe, and studies have shown just how powerful community can be in resolving addiction. In 1978, Canadian psychologist Bruce K. Alexander conducted the famous Rat Park experiment and revolutionized the way we understand drug addiction.[8]

In Alexander's experiment, the social rats had a choice to drink either tap water or a morphine solution, as compared to rats in solitary confinement with the same choices. He found that the social rats resisted the morphine, preferring the water, while the solitary, caged rats ingested much larger doses of the morphine solution—about 19 times more than Rat Park rats. Even caged rats fed nothing but morphine water for 57 days, when moved to Rat Park, chose plain water, voluntarily going through withdrawal. No matter what they tried, Alexander and his team produced nothing that resembled addiction in rats that were housed in the Rat Park.

Based on the study, the team concluded that drugs themselves do not cause addictions, but rather addiction is caused by feelings of isolation, loneliness, hopelessness, and lack of control based on unsatisfactory living conditions. What this tells us is that, even in animals, community is the prevention and the treatment for self-abuse. (Many argue that 12 Step programs enjoy the persistent success that they do because they offer community.)

*When these things are finally granted to us, a wave of recognition rises that we have lived without this love, this acknowledgment, and the support of this village all of our lives.*

— FRANCIS WELLER, AUTHOR OF *THE WILD EDGE OF SORROW*

In so many ways, our health is intertwined with our experience of human connection. The science tells us social isolation leads to chronic, deadly inflammation.[9] So why, then, if we are wired for connectivity and community, do so many of us find ourselves feeling lost and alone, suffering the mental and physical consequences of the "community wound"?

I became aware of the pulsing, raw nature of this wound at a workshop when I did an exercise that had me look into the eyes of a stranger for 2 minutes. Tears flowed within the first 30 seconds. This is the near-universal experience of this kind of intimacy because we are all wounded in community. But the simple connection with a stranger can show us how little is required to take off our masks and feel what is missing, to see ourselves in another, and to have deep empathy wash over us.

The community wound is a deep one for me. Fiercely independent, I made my mission self-sufficiency from an early age. Asking for advice, guidance, support, or counsel was a form of weakness, something for "others" to indulge and for me to remain squarely on the dispensing end of. I didn't know that I was protecting a need so intense that to expose it to the light of day would bring me into contact with a deep wellspring of unmet needs and grief.

I have found a deep healing of this wound through my daughters' Waldorf school, where parents devoted to the teachings of Rudolf Steiner, visionary founder of anthroposophical theory, gather in service of their children's spirits. I was ready to truly embrace this community because I'd had soul sisters who were by my side throughout my many Dark Nights, readying me to receive more love in my life.

## Separation or Connection?

My friend Charles Eisenstein, author of *The More Beautiful World Our Hearts Know Is Possible* and other soul-expanding texts, has an explanation for why we may all be suffering so, when he refers to our disconnection as originating in what he calls the Story of Separation. The Story of Separation is the Cartesian story of dualism: the mechanical body and its discrete companion, mind. It's a story of humanity as separate from others, the environment, God, and our souls. In this story, we harbor the collective pain that this separation and its myriad consequences and outgrowths create.

Eisenstein calls for us to move into a different story, one he calls the Story of Interbeing, in which there is an intelligent universe based on cooperativity and co-creation, not dominance. It is a story of a more feminine power that fits perfectly with ancient wisdom, one that demolishes false boundaries and illuminates the interconnected systems within the body, between body and environment, and even between ourselves and our divine power.

We must all choose which Story to believe in. Are you, as Alan Watts would say is the dominant view, an "accidental microorganism infesting a minute globular rock that revolves about an unimportant star on the outer fringe of one of the minor galaxies," seeking dominion over nature, over the bad guys, and over your malfunctioning and faulty body parts? Or are you a being with unique gifts here to uplift the experience of others through your own connectedness to the spirit within and around you in a web of conscious, intelligent, and purposeful energy?

It's time to get back to a felt experience of our humanity, and the first sign of readiness is the ache of that connection's strain, its absence. So many of us are looking for that one person who will guide us in this effort, but it may very well be that we have to do it together. Vietnamese Buddhist teacher Thich Nhat Hanh reminds us that community is the guru of the future. He means by this that the unique alchemy of our togetherness will ultimately serve to empower, heal, and guide us. The guru is not the expert, and the guru may not even simply be "within." Instead, the guru is the web, the union, the sum greater than the parts, and it may be the case that we cannot heal fully without the sacredness of this reality informing our every moment.

For this reason and more, we have created the Vital Life Project as a companion to this book, a community movement that creates a safe space for the consciousness of self-reclamation. In the project, we move through one step a month of a felt shift in physical health, so as to awaken the innate healing response, with the energy of a group powering the momentum of change.

## MEDICAL TREATMENT: RAISING AWARENESS AROUND OUR CHOICES

When we think of relationships, we think of people in communication. Our relationships are with everything around us, including systems, institutions, and elements of the natural world. We all have a relationship to the dominant medical system. For most of us, our habitual response to medical treatment has been driven by fear and reactivity. We have outsourced our trust to authorities who reflect back to us a harrowing tale of our health prospects and a new normal of chronic disease. We have lost our essential selves in our collective love affair with our intellects and the promise of dominating the world, nature, and our bodies.

And there is a subconscious messaging that gets imbedded every time you run to a doctor or fill a prescription: the message is that you are somehow broken and beyond self-help. When you need to "fix" your physical signs and symptoms, behavior, mood, or mind, you are saying *no* to yourself and seeking others who are going to help you experience yourself as a victim of your own body.

But there's another way you can embrace, and it involves *knowing*, not thinking.

Reconnect to your inner compass to come into deeper contact with what your soul knows to be true: that your *response* to illness, from a place of deep faith in the body, is your best treatment, and that mindful living is your best intervention. That given, each and every interaction with the medical system deserves a conscious assessment: What does this express about my beliefs around health and the body? In the era of consensus medicine, it is imperative to hold every assumption about conventional interventions up to the harsh light of truth.

It comes down to this: if you want to feel strong, free, and real, you've got to make health care decisions that reflect the consciousness you are looking to embody. Don't be the devoted yogi with a prescribing M.D. on speed dial for every scary symptom. You must choose whether you believe that your body has an innate wisdom, a vitalism that guides its natively harmonious performance. That illness is evidence of imbalance somewhere—physically, mentally, spiritually, interpersonally, nutritionally—and that it is an invitation to engage change in the service of balance.

The other choice is that we are born with our destiny set by our genes. That our bodies are finely calibrated machines that are prone to break down, requiring repair, servicing, and maintenance. That "the science is settled" (about *anything*). That doctors are beyond reproach. That it is better to be safe than sorry.

You cannot have it both ways: either you are aligned with your body and supporting it, or you are managing and fighting it because you and those around you are scared into reactivity. Because every time you open that pill bottle, you are saying *nope, you don't got this* to your body. You are enforcing a message of oppression by a system that says *feeling* is dangerous—feeling anything—when you know full well that feeling is where your true power lies.

---

*All illness is created first in the mind. All of life is first a thought. Thoughts are like magnets, they draw things. Thoughts may not always be obvious as in "I am going to contract a terrible disease." A thought may be subtle, "I am not worthy of living."*

— NEALE DONALD WALSCH, *CONVERSATIONS WITH GOD*

---

## Pharma-Free Living

So how do you do this, practically, in the real world? What does the person with insulin resistance, diabetes, chronic headaches/

migraines, gastroesophageal reflux disease, or allergies do, for example? What do you do when you get a bad cold, torn muscle, or upset stomach and want to use symptom suppressors from your local drugstore?

Here's my advice: make your decision for treatment with *all* available information. I believe first and foremost in informed consent. I understand that it is not my role to tell anyone else what to do, but it *is* my role to reflect back to my patients and readers their own held beliefs so that in times of struggle, they can avoid succumbing to the horror story their mind (doctor, uncle, media) is telling them.

Informed consent requires that you know more than what the very corporate purveyors of a product would like you to know. More than what coopted regulatory bodies like the Food and Drug Administration and Centers for Disease Control would like you to know. More than media, the last bastion of checks and balances, now lost, would like you to know. Only then can you get free from the "better-safe-than-sorry" default mechanism that has been guiding your every medical choice.

In Appendix B, I offer a natural medicine toolkit to help you support your body's recalibration around stressors, conflicts, and detox. In so many cases, symptoms appearing as recognizable infections are here to help us sloooow down and improve basic self-care. Having these tools on hand can help soothe the reflexive fear that can arise, and also appease the belief that we need to "take something" in order to get better.

---

### Resetter: Lucy

It's true: we really are the experts in matters of our own body and health. After completing the program, my anxiety is *way* down, I'm almost completely weaned off my 30-year usage of Prozac, and I'm in touch with a feeling of inner peace.

As I move forward, I plan to listen to information as it comes my way but then check in to see if it resonates with my experience or it feels like someone else's "should." Lastly, I truly believe we are all on this planet doing the best we can. Eating real food, focusing on positive thoughts, and surrounding myself with supportive people are all part of my wellness plan moving forward.

---

## Pharma-Free Parenting: The How-To

I have a pharma-free household, and my daughters have never been to a doctor or emergency room for an illness. That said, having trained in functional medicine, I spent years trying to negotiate with them to choke back supplement tinctures of fatty acids, probiotics, minerals, and herbs. But soon, after one too many battles and a growing sense that I was overly attached to their cooperation in this arena, I realized that the more I pushed their vitamins, the more I was sending a message to them that their bodies needed these vitamins and were incomplete without them.

And so we have settled on energy medicine. My two daughters take flower remedies and homeopathy without resistance when needed, and they are in charge of self-administering.

I couldn't have been more inspired to have the opportunity to ask Master Mingtong Gu,[10] during my first Qigong training, about how and what this powerful practice can offer children. If conventional medicine is the push-pull, Newtonian, body-as-machine model of health, Qigong is the opposite, a nonlinear, quantum, soul-as-body model of health. This ancient practice—visualization, sound, and slow movement—allows each person to engage in radical self-healing of stuck energy and cellular memories of trauma—also known as *illness*!

Here are Mingtong's recommendations for bringing this energetic practice to your family:

- **Model body confidence.** When a child trips and falls, what's the first thing they do? They check for your reaction. If you freak out, so do they. If you reflect confidence in their resilience, they get up and keep running! Use phrases like "Your body can handle this . . . it knows exactly what to do . . . let me help you listen to what your body is saying."

- **Stay with the body.** Help your child embody by asking them where they feel what they feel. They can point to it, describe it, and share what it's like. You can even ask them to imagine that they are traveling within their own body. What does it look like in there? What do they see?

- **Bring the love where it's needed.** The inner smile meditation is exactly what it sounds like: the practice of bringing the energy of a smile to where it hurts. This is the foundational practice of moving toward, not away from the pain, struggle, and challenge. Being with it, even loving it. Teach your child: imagine a warm light traveling inward from your smiling face toward the heart and then to every organ and cell in the body, leaving each smiling. This simple practice can act as the foundation for a lifetime of embracing what is.

- **Meditate together.** Lachi is one of the foundational meditative practices of Qigong; Mingtong demonstrates it in a video you can find on YouTube.[11] Kids love meditating! And they love chanting. So spend a few minutes feeling the "chi ball" and chanting Hao-la, which means "All is well . . . getting better" or Kai-her for expansion and gathering. Invite them to bring this activated chi ball to where it hurts in their body to move that stuck energy.

If symptoms are reframed, not as a nuisance, not as a problem, but as an expression of the body that requires attention, support, and focused intention, *self-empowerment, self-confidence, and personal trust* are amplified. These are the keys to unlocking an entirely different relationship to health and healing—a more beautiful story. Parents have a precious opportunity to shift the consciousness of the next generation through these simple practices so we can get to the heart of our true work as parents: helping our children feel their emotions.

In service of this goal, my daughter Sofia and I published an illustrated children's book called *A Time for Rain* to support parents in teaching the power of emotions—not just happiness—to heal, and to link us together in purposeful harmony.

## Travel Tip for Medical Treatment

**Heal yourself first**. Our children's illnesses can be expressions of our own unprocessed shadow material, as they hold our grief and fears for us. This is why I always recommend to parents that their own healing be prioritized. It is the most powerful thing you can do for your children and will also free you to be fully present to their spiritual development. Author Dr. Shefali Tsabary, who wrote *The Awakened Family: How to Raise Empowered, Resilient, and Conscious Children*, would argue that our primary responsibility as parents is to guide and honor our children's spirits.

## YOUR WORK LIFE: WHAT'S YOUR PURPOSE?

So you've performed a security clearance on your family and intimate relationships, you've readied your mindset to ride the waves of your health challenges, and then you wake up one day and realize you cannot go to your office job ever again. Not for one more minute.

My patients come to me working jobs in conventional systems like schools, financial institutions, and hospitals, and they leave as healers, artists, and conscious entrepreneurs. Over and over again, I have observed that as we wake up, the first impulse we have is to pay it forward. To serve. To give of ourselves and our now-full cup. To have a sense of purpose. They want to feel that their life has value, that the work they do demonstrates that value. So they create the life and job they never knew they could before.

It's not that this sense of fulfillment cannot be found in a 9-to-5 job. It is, of course, possible to bring the consciousness of joy to any life circumstance. It's just that most of us do well to align our daily activities with what brings us joy before we can consistently bring joy to our daily activities. As Neale Donald Walsch writes in *Conversations with God*:

If you believe you are a "person who supports his family at all costs, even sacrificing his own happiness," then you should *love* your hard work in life since it *facilitates* your statement of your Self as you have chosen. You should not complain how hard you work to support your family.

If you see yourself as a "woman who works at a job she hates in order to meet responsibilities as she sees them," then you should love your hard job, for it totality supports your self-image.

We can love everything the moment we understand what we are doing and why. No one does anything they do not want to do.[12]

It often turns out that the jobs we choose from our child-self wounds never really fulfill us. The achievement/productivity program is a fear-based defensive structure, and this explains why there's no amount of achievement that ever really leaves us feeling full. This is also why, as you allow these structures to fall apart and courageously endure the shock waves of financial concerns—the "what will everyone think" concerns and the free fall sense of lost identity—you will finally begin to have experiences that actually bring you deep fulfillment and also happen to magnetize prosperity and ease.

The Japanese have a word for this: *ikigai*. This refers to a concept that means "a reason for being." It is a mindset that is at the source of value in one's life or the things that make one's life worthwhile. Each individual's ikigai is personal to them and specific to their lives, values, and beliefs. It reflects your inner self and faithfully expresses that, while simultaneously creating a mental state in which you feel at ease. Activities that allow one to feel *ikigai* are never forced by obligation, but rather are spontaneous and always undertaken willingly, giving you a sense of satisfaction and of meaning to life. In the culture of Okinawa, *ikigai* is thought of as "a reason to get up in the morning."

In Western terms, we might think of *ikigai* relating directly to having a sense of energy flow, to tapping into our primal life force energy that comes available when you're truly living our purpose. The Hindu term is *shakti*, derived from the Sanskrit "to be able."

This primal energy is *always* in there, waiting to be accessed. But we have locked it up at the command of our productivity-oriented systems, and we pretend it doesn't exist. We go to our jobs, we check off the to-do list, we contribute our small but significant part to planetary death and destruction, and we turn a blind eye to all that might provoke too much *feeling*. And then we wonder why we are so tired!

So here's the question: What are you doing to tap into your life force energy? What in your life really turns you on? If your answer is nothing, perhaps your soul is saying no—and you are calling that *fatigue*.

Here's what one of my online participants said after completing the program and making major changes in her life.

---

### Resetter: Nina

Emotionally, I feel more even, steady. I started tapering the Cipralex this weekend, and even though this part will come with greater challenges, I feel ready to face them. One of these is the decision I made to resign from my stressful job with a long commute and make solid plans to start a private practice in my town. This is part of my radical self-care plan: no more 10-plus hours per week in the car, no more high-stress meetings and cases that blow up like garbage fires, no more trying to take care of so many people in the agency. My focus continues to be (now more than ever): take excellent care of my young daughter and myself—the rest will take care of itself.

---

## Energy Drains

Fatigue lends itself perfectly to the multiple-narrative model of medicine. Psychiatry views fatigue as a brain-based imbalance or deficiency likely responsive to a stimulant or antidepressant. Functional medicine views fatigue more as stemming from bodily causes: hypothyroidism, $B_{12}$ deficiency or poor methylation, adrenal fatigue, or general mitochondrial dysfunction, where low nutrient supply and abundant toxicant exposure impair energy-making cellular centers.

While I do believe in healing the body first to clarify matters of spirit, I also urge you to get curious and search for the meaning of fatigue in your life, rather than accepting it at face value. What is your tiredness telling you? Is your fatigue a sign of incomplete alignment with self and/or a given activity, even your chosen vocation?

For example, I hate food shopping. I think my soul knows there is something wrong with driving to a building and exchanging paper for food I didn't procure. I yawn all the way to Whole Foods. Every. Time. But at my desk, doing what I love most, I feel like I'm plugged into a live wire, I have so much energy.

When you feel tired, irritable, or checked out, ask if there's something you need to see there. Are you doing what is in your best and highest interest in your life and chosen vocation? If not, how can you break out? What can you reexamine? What is it that you are saying no to and how can you generate the conditions for a yes?

## Travel Tip for Work: Go with the Flow

You don't have to jump on LinkedIn in search of a value-driven new job or position. There are actually no big decisions to be made when you are in the flow of your own awakened self. The only thing you have to do is keep clear (remember the practices in Part II!) and re-dedicate yourself to self-care every day so you will be able to inquire into, receive, and recognize the invitations, opportunities, and "signs" that a new vocation is in order, one that connects you with your new "reason for being."

## ALICIA'S STORY: EYES WIDE OPEN

Alicia was first medicated for college-related anxiety and came to me at age 33 determined to taper off medication, stating that it never felt aligned with her belief system. Through the Reset, she resolved chronic irritable bowel syndrome symptoms as well as nightly asthma for which she had used an inhaler since 4th grade. After having attempted to taper repeatedly and failed without a Reset, this time she finally got free.

She wrote:

Today marks two months since the last time I pulled the bottle of Lexapro out of my refrigerator, pulled the liquid up to the .1 mark on the syringe, and let the toxic substance slide down the back of my throat. I don't know how all this time just went by without a blink, but here we are . . .

This journey has been one of the hardest, yet most beautiful things I have ever done in my life. I have learned so much and I cannot quiet the burning feeling in my gut that's constantly pulling me to a higher purpose. The calling is only getting louder as the days after quitting the medication grow farther and farther away.

Trying to satisfy that feeling, I explored all these avenues that were seemingly in the realm I wanted to be. I approached each of these avenues with a sense of apprehension because I somewhat knew they weren't quite right even before I started exploring. These were the avenues where the universe never sent me a clear sign telling me *yes*. They were the type of avenues that my current "career self" would say was the "right thing to do" . . . the same career that grew while being medicated. This approach just wasn't going to fly now that I was awake. My creative self who had been asleep for over 10 years woke back up and said, *Sorry—we aren't doing this again*, and I knew I needed to listen.

Over time, two visions presented themselves to me that I know I need to follow, one that I think involves you in some way . . .

In the midst of the very tumultuous times during the taper, I saw these glimmers of light and I started writing them down for fear that my fogged mind would forget. As these thoughts started to accumulate on the page, I realized that I needed to do something with them. I needed to be sure that the others going through this pain knew that there *would* be moments of peace. In the middle of the night I awoke to a vision of a book. The cover art, the story, the chapters. I grabbed my notebook and started writing down everything I saw because I was again afraid that my seemingly hijacked mind would not remember. At this point, I was still tapering and was afraid to "formally" start writing until I was through to the other side. Finally, one Friday morning after I had stopped the medicine, I took the handcuffs off myself and just starting writing it. I have no idea if I will ever do anything with it, but I followed this calling because it was impossible to ignore the pull toward it.

A second vision came to me just recently, again in the middle of the night while I was sleeping. Throughout my taper journey, my soul became alive again, just like so many of us who have gone through it. I am back to the person I was, but with a knowledge money can't buy. This movement toward allowing people to see that the power of their health is in their own hands fuels me. Your work around letting people see that life without medication is truly where we are meant to be lights me up inside. I know firsthand what that feels like and it's incredibly empowering. It's also incredibly hard because you want to shout it from the rooftop and assume everyone will follow, but I've learned that you can only truly help those who are ready and open.

The vision I saw that night was supporting your movement in some way. It's not quite clear to me how that support will manifest itself, and I am not sure that you even need or want my support, but because that vision presented itself to me so clearly, I figured I should once again take the handcuffs off and do something about it, so here I am . . .

I finally sat down to write you this note this morning, and I saw a very timely e-mail arrive in my inbox about a very similar subject . . . I just looked to the sky and laughed. This universe is truly divine if we just learn to surrender to it. I am grateful for the 11 years that I have worked hard and built a business career because it certainly served its purpose and brought me to where I am in this moment, but I realize how important it is that my work also comes from my soul, just as I had envisioned it when I was younger.

ൠ

## What's Next . . .

In our final chapter, we will explore what it's like to live as an awakened adult, your childself healed and all aspects of your new life aligned and flowing for the greatest harmony and ease. Here's where you get the tools you'll need for a full lifetime of accessing the field of possibility and feeling the mystery, awe, and joy of life.

Chapter 10

# FAITH: TRUST IN A GRAND DESIGN

*What will be, will be well—for what is, is well.*

— WALT WHITMAN

By this final chapter, you've gotten the message: health is not simply about meds or no meds; it's about answering the question that your symptoms are asking. Once you've done that, you can choose to shed the aspects of your life that are keeping you sick, stuck, and out of alignment. The ongoing work of this transformation process is one of integration, and it requires that you live life from a new mindset and align important elements of your lifestyle with that mindset.

In this chapter, I am going to focus on one more phase of your transformation: integrating a spiritual viewpoint into your daily life. Living an awakening life day in and day out requires faith, a sense that the design of your journey is intelligent. In this chapter, I will share how you can facilitate, induce, and support having trust and faith that you are being held by something greater for a life of flow, expansion, and ease.

Importantly, I am not a spiritual guru. I am not here to pretend to give you some kind of map that I've divined. I hope to share what I've learned on the way and what I've learned from the many

I've walked alongside through the Dark Night awakening process. Put these considerations in your toolkit and know that you will be attracted to exactly what you need now that you are clear enough to perceive it.

## A DISTORTED VIEW OF SPIRITUALITY

Our Western paradigm of what is "normal" disallows any sense of true spirituality in our culture. Psychiatry especially does this, imposing medical standards that define what is real and what is unreal in our human experience. Psychiatry dismisses any sensory experience that exists outside the mind and manifests as visual or auditory images, labeling that experience *hallucination*. Not real.

---

*The worldview created by traditional Western science and dominating our culture is, in its most rigorous form, incompatible with any notion of spirituality.*

— STANISLAV GROF, M.D.

---

In my training, I learned clinical, diagnostic terms like "magical thinking" to pedantically dismiss any flourishes of wonderment, "delusions of reference" to coldly malign any experience of meaning or synchronicity, and even "grandiosity" if you might deign to think too much of yourself.

When human behavior is medicalized and we participate in that medical system, we are tacitly consenting to what we will uphold as normal and abnormal, acceptable and unacceptable, sick and healthy. Some behaviors are unacceptable; some are not. And conforming to these expectations—even through force and involuntary submission, retention, and medication—is essential to reinforcing what is considered normal. Those who are not performing their expected part in the machinery of this system are deemed less or nonfunctional (the quantification of which, psychiatry assigns a numerical value based on the Global Assessment of Functioning metric scale).

But what if being "functional" requires buying into an entire matrix of illusions, many of which require a total divorce from one's own soul?

In Chapter 1, I shared my belief that those labeled mentally ill are the canaries in this coal mine, those whose bodies, minds, and spirits are exquisitely sensitive to all that is off, amiss, misaligned, and divergent from truth. Given that understanding, illnesses can be seen as a special invitation to wake up, to embody, and to move through a Dark Night, a tight passage, shedding one more artificial skin, revealing a layer closer to an unfettered experience of being, of freedom, and of joy.

In this view, those who still believe that we are simply, as philosopher Alan Watts says in describing the dominant view, *flesh robots on a dead rock, spinning out in the middle of nowhere*—are, in fact, *the ones hallucinating*. They believe that the natural world is an indifferent backdrop subject to random forces that we must shield ourselves from. They still embrace Newtonian physics—linear cause and effect, what you get out is what you put in, push-pull hydraulics—rather than the subtler, nonlinear quantum processes. Quantum physics introduces all manner of uncomfortable concepts to those fixated on the delusional belief that there is an objective, quantifiable, measurable reality of known variables that predictably governs a nonsentient universe.

Consider that *that* linear, dualistic belief is a collectively held hallucination. Those who have had mystical experiences know it is but an illusion that the natural world needs to be managed and controlled. Instead, they know that we *emerge* from the complexity of beingness on this planet, and that there really is no objective good or bad, and perhaps no objective anything at all.

Here is the question: What if your so-called mental illness is a sign of sanity, an opportunity to awaken and express your gifts, while those embracing the orthodox beliefs and behaviors are more likely than you to meet the criteria for mental illness?

This was certainly true for Dr. Joan Borysenko, a beautiful, brilliant author and visionary in the field of psychoneuroimmunology and mind-body medicine. I recently heard her talk at a workshop where she shared her remarkable story of childhood "mental illness":

how at age 10, she experienced an alternate reality, what psychiatry would label as psychosis and OCD. After several months, she recovered almost overnight through a profound spiritual experience that changed her perception of life. A few moments of contact with the soul—what she calls her inner physician or authentic Self—provided her with the inner strength and guidance she needed to heal. That fleeting glimpse of her soul during a dark time marked her early spiritual evolution that contributed directly to the prismatic being she is today.[1]

## SPIRITUAL EMERGENCE/Y

Shamanic lineages better understand people considered as hallucinating to be special or gifted. Defined broadly as an ancient healing tradition, *shamanism* is thought to grant access to a realm of consciousness that healers can bring their subjects into and through. With soul retrieval, cleansing, and even saying deep, soul-level good-byes to deceased loved ones, shamans have an esoteric tool kit.

I recently learned of the work of Malidoma Somé, a West African shaman, through documentary filmmaker Emma Bragdon of IMHU (Integrative Mental Health for You).[2] Somé speaks of *spiritual emergency*, which is when a person is overwhelmed and disoriented by spiritual experiences. Somé believes that people who are given labels of serious mental disorders are sensitives who need training and support to become the healers and psychic mediums they are meant to be. They are the wounded healers.[3]

---

*In the West [we] are not trained in how to deal or even taught to acknowledge the existence of psychic phenomena, the spiritual world. In fact, psychic abilities are denigrated. When energies from the spiritual world emerge in a Western psyche, that individual is completely unequipped to integrate them or even recognize what is happening. The result can be terrifying.*

— MALIDOMA SOMÉ

---

Knowledge of our psychic connections with spirits is not entirely unknown in our Western paradigm. Over one hundred years ago, William James, M.D., considered the father of American psychology, collaborated with researchers of psychic phenomena.[4] He said we must research psychic phenomena and consider it as having a vital role in the challenges of being human. This message is but a faint echo in today's research and practices within psychology.

Fortunately, once we become aware that our experience is a hallucination, that hallucination dissolves. In the case of the dominant belief system—the most collectively shared hallucination—dissolution is called *awakening*. When we awaken, we become aware that the story we've been telling ourselves is a story, nothing more.

Call it living in the matrix, call it hallucinating, or the illusion—if you live life according to what mainstream media, government, and appointed authorities say is so, there may come a time when you crack and are labeled with ADHD, generalized anxiety, major depression, schizophrenia, or bipolar disorder. You will be told *you* are the sick one, that something is wrong with your inbuilt hard-ware. The figurative bone will be pointed at you and the collective will support your containment, restraint, and oppression to keep the infrastructure of the illusion intact.

But the mortar is cracking. Too many of us have felt the truth that is spirituality. To be infused with spirit. To feel your own soul. To stop and inspire, breathe, and understand that without the *entire* ecosystem of beingness on this planet, you yourself are nothing. Once you have felt the fearlessness of this faith, you can never be controlled again, and you are finally free.

---

*Faith is a state of openness or trust. To have faith is like when you trust yourself to the water. You don't grab hold of the water when you swim, because if you do you will become stiff and tight in the water, and sink. You have to relax . . . the attitude of faith is to let go, and become open to truth, whatever it might turn out to be.*

— ALAN WATTS

---

## WHAT IT MEANS TO BE WOKE

Today, in spite of the dominant belief system, we are in the midst of a spirituality zeitgeist. There is a New Age shop selling crystals and tarot cards in every town, you can be shamed for never having done yoga, and everyone has a "healer." But what does it mean to be "woke"? Certainly it can't simply mean you have adequate disposable income to spend on the trappings of Eastern-inspired practices?

The path of my own spiritual awakening was anything but predictable. As I've shared, I was an atheist from the moment I could make up my own mind on the matter, and remained a belligerent one who thought belief in a greater power was for weak people who needed a bedtime story to ease them to sleep at night.

My path was filled with breakdowns and breakthroughs, intense and seemingly relentless self-work, much of which led me to prioritize ease, pleasure, and doing less. The words of my mentor, Nicholas Gonzalez, reflect the dilemma I and so many others confront when moving from nonbelief to a greater understanding. He wrote in a letter to me, "I approach atheism the way I approach adolescent acne, as a phase many go through that is meant to be outgrown, discarded, and forgotten. Unfortunately too many 'smart' people stay stuck in adolescent levels of spiritual understanding, which limits them in their personal lives and precludes, in our particular profession, physicians from becoming truly healing."

In the West, it seems we have a choice of two camps: atheism or denominational religion that relegates spirituality to the nonphysical and nonmaterial. But there is, in fact, another option. Another path could be a truly spiritual one, one in which you find emergent perfection in all that is and defer to a cosmic design, a great meta-organism, of which we are all contributing cellular components— parts of an interdependent whole that is, paradoxically, reliant on each cell having intact cell wall boundaries!

The effort toward shedding layers of illusory "what-you-see-is-all-there-is" reality is the spiritual path. In this process, you identify the feeling of true freedom and realize your illusory self was just an elaborate compensation for the wound. Once you are able to do that, you're free to align with the adult consciousness of clarity, strength, and intimacy with emotional states from a witness-consciousness perspective, understanding that you are the universe itself in the act of creation.

But with your first mystical experience can come an attachment to that feeling of expansion, light, and union. Through spiritual bypassing, many on paths of self-development and metaphysical exploration ignore and dismiss the role of painful emotions in the complete human experience.

Robert Augustus Masters, often cited as an expert on the ways people use spirituality to avoid taking responsibility for their actions, wrote a book with that same title, *Spiritual Bypassing.* He also invites us to welcome our shadow elements into the fold of spirituality. And he cautions that any kind of righteousness about one's spirituality is just another form of shadow material. Deep spirituality is relinquishing the need to escape anything or run toward anything—it is rather, accepting what is, and then exploring what is for personal meaning. He writes: "Cutting through spiritual bypassing means turning toward the painful, disfigured, ostracized, unwanted, or otherwise disowned aspects of ourselves and cultivating as much intimacy as possible with them."

---

### Resetter: Risa

Five years ago my body was so broken by stress and a tick-borne infection that I was incontinent, couldn't follow a TV program, and struggled to read my child's kindergarten book. I was even being tested for early onset Alzheimer's. Today, after completing the Reset program, my brain is growing stronger, my cognitive functioning is improving, and I'm able to accomplish things I couldn't before. I feel joy, hope, and energy pouring out of me into the universe, and feel that I'm part of something big, something positive that I've never felt before. This is not just "alternative," "hippie" stuff. These are real changes that are happening, and it's incredibly powerful and empowering.

---

## BUILDING YOUR NEW LIFE: TIME TO MAN/WOMAN UP

There comes a moment in every awakening process when it's time to take the wheel and man/woman up to owning and creating your life. Not the *you* that you were, but the real, *adult* you that is now being born. You need to become the boss of your experience, because in the quantum reality you are now aligned with, you create what you want with your beliefs and intention—you are responsible.

When you have moved through the *feeling* experience of letting those powerful forces mobilize (this comes in waves of intense windows), you can begin to relate to your childself from a place of adult authority. You begin the lifelong process of parenting yourself in ways that you were likely never parented. This is self-mastery.

You choose to stop running around life as a grown child: entitled, reactive, and playing out dynamics that should have been left in the distant past. That's where our victim stories take root—because we were belittled, diminished, shamed, hurt, and neglected at a time when we needed protection and unconditional love, at a time when we needed to be told, as the popular TV show host Fred Rogers ("Mr. Rogers") attempted to tell his audience, we are "just fine the way we are."

When you begin to heal these wounds, you must leave the victim mindset behind. Remember: that's how conventional medicine gets its hooks in you; it reinforces that victim mentality that you are powerless to do anything but fill a prescription. It feels good and validating, but it ultimately keeps you arrested as a child, never to become an empowered and initiated adult.

When I made a major move in my life in a grand effort to consciously construct my adult identity in the aftermath of a decimating spiritual awakening, I was given an important opportunity to see that no amount of fixing the outside makes the inside okay. Turns out it wasn't New York City that was making me a neurotically driven workaholic productivity addict. That was all an inside job.

Somehow, in the wake of my relocation, I spent the first three months focusing on what *still* wasn't quite right in the grand scheme of my life despite the glaciers and boulders I had moved (and watched move) to get to this place. I focused on what cords were still hanging on. Who still needed to move? What needed to fit in place that wasn't quite there? It was a list I perseverated on like the CEO of an unprofitable company. My lighthouse was scanning, perpetuating the "I'll feel good when . . ." illusion that my okay-ness lies in arranging life just so, rather than in finally gathering up the parts of me I was still habitually running from.

One day, I'd had enough. Enough of my scarcity mentality. My negativity. The white-noise hum of discomfort that attachment to future outcomes produces. And honestly, I'd had enough of not being able to *feel* all that was right, the perfection of all things I'd come to appreciate through my incredibly intricate and impossible-to-foresee process of dissolution and rebuilding.

And then my best friend, Tahra, an intuitive, psychic medium, and all-around soul-accountability partner, said, "If you don't have something in your life, it's because you don't want it." She was right; I was addicted to being a victim, even choosing victimhood rather than confronting the programs of control that arose from that victim posture.

Here are two strategies you can employ to become the boss of your life and ensure that you stay on the path of adult empowerment:

## Strategy #1: Accept Discomfort and Stop Complaining

We Westerners tend to be more negative than those in the East, complaining about things our Eastern counterparts wouldn't even think of giving negative lip service to. In India, a country I've visited and where I've witnessed life firsthand, people have very little to be objectively pleased about through the lens of Western materialism, so it's shocking to find a surplus of everyday joy, generosity, and gratitude.

It's possible that our Western negativity reflects a desire to feel whole. Unlike people in third world countries, we are feeling the pain of what is invisibly missing; in fact, one of the roots of the word *complain* is the Latin word for *grieve*. We feel, even if unconsciously, that community, a connection to the earth, and intergenerational wisdom are undergoing extinction. We have gaping wounds that we are stuffing with secondary satisfactions. We want for more all the time, thinking that what we get—house, job, lover, money—will stop the ache within, only to find that it doesn't. It therefore makes sense that we would be striving, ever striving to fix the problem, which requires focusing on the problem—and complaining endlessly.

I choose to see our Western negativity bias as our *discomfort with discomfort*.

Stopping this cycle requires expanding our comfort zone to include challenging emotions like sadness, grief, and anguish. To stop seeking the magic pill and final quick fix, but instead embrace nuance and meaning. There is a profound solace in the exploration of right timing and purposeful design in this human experience.

If you can translate your mess into meaning, you have a chance to free yourself and actually feel the mess rather than simply bypass or fix it. This is not the same as being happy about things your mind is telling you are wrong. It's not a whitewashing. It's allowing the bass tones to coexist in the symphony of treble notes. In this way, you can better embrace seemingly negative emotions as part of a larger process. In fact, a 1,300-person study revealed that accepting negative emotions rather than suppressing, fighting, or otherwise papering them over led to the experience of fewer negative emotions![5]

In sum, if you accept your negative emotions, you'll think fewer negative thoughts, because feeling bad is less likely to grab the mind's roving lighthouse lantern. Said another way, when you stop fighting what you are feeling—scared, alone, abandoned, angry— you spend less time focusing on what's wrong in your life that needs fixing, and complain less. Only through this portal of acceptance do you have the opportunity to finally drop into the vast okay-ness of it all and truly live an awakened life of faith.

## Strategy #2: Own Your Power

When I began my "adultification" process, my family therapist told me to sit down and pen my ideal daily schedule. *What?* But what about the 10,000 variables I was trying to accommodate and the logistics and the finances and the . . . *Just sit down and create it,* she said.

And I did, even though it was much harder than one would imagine. This is because the norm is to focus most of our energy on what we don't want, not on what could be. Once I made that shift and focused on what I wanted, the possibilities I'd written down manifested into reality to create what had seemed impossible: specifically, family dynamics lining up and a flow unfolding to usher me into my best life. All I had done was exercise my authority to create.

Here are some essential guidelines to support you through your own adultification process:

*To own your power, try putting your victim story into words.* Our lives are defined by patterns. There are ways in which we struggle and suffer at the hands of others, over and over again. Whatever it is that keeps happening to you, put it into one sentence, write it down, and see what themes emerge. Are you left out? Do you feel invisible? Do you feel always unlucky? Are people always taking advantage of you? Odds are, the origin of these stories is early in your life when you developed such a belief about yourself as a way to make sense out of your childhood experience.

A recent example in my life was that I recorded a very vulnerable voice text to a family member with whom I have had years of tension and ledger-like dynamics. We both felt aggrieved that the other never "showed up" in the way we wanted, each keeping an abacus on the other's life performance. In my voice memo, I expressed fears that I have and a need I feel to be seen and accepted.

I sent the text and went on with my life. Two weeks went by with no response. I talked to friends about how expected that was. *Of course he didn't respond,* I complained. *He's so self-absorbed and unable to deal with me or communicate consciously.* I felt victimized, again. Until I checked and realized that the text had never actually gone through. That little red exclamation point indicted me, and I was forced to recognize that I had actually created a situation—albeit, unconsciously—where I could continue to feel like a victim. When he responded only a few hours later, I was forced to experience the discomfort I felt in response to his openness and receptivity.

In this situation, I had an opportunity to see my shadow at work and to accept the vulnerability in no longer being a victim, in dropping that story. Instead, I could move into a place of personal responsibility for my part in a painful relationship that has an opportunity to transform, and compassion for the fear that kept me stuck in a patterned experience I hated every minute of.

There are myriad manifestation practices out there for developing the life you deserve, and for having an experience of yourself liberated from old patterns, conditioning, and the role you played as a child meeting your parents' (and other authorities') needs. The Law of Attraction, Reality Transurfing, and other methods all tell the same story: get clear on the inside, leverage the quantum power of emotions like gratitude, and the outside will show you that the impossible is indeed possible. All you need to do is claim it.

---

*By turning toward your painful emotions, especially those you tend to label as negative, you will start to feel a more embodied sense of wholeness, a sense of internalized reunion and communion. Instead of abandoning or trying to transcend what is unwanted, disowned, ostracized, or otherwise cast aside in you, you can include it in your being, intimately, until it is no longer a distant "it" but rather a reclaimed you.*

— ROBERT AUGUSTUS MASTERS, *EMOTIONAL INTIMACY*

---

## MOVING BEYOND LIMITATIONS

Here's the big reveal: Once you claim your true adult power, you begin to move beyond the limited metrics of a quantifiable energy reserve. You begin to enter your flow.

You've probably heard of the concept of "flow" and think it's synonymous with "success." It's not. Accessing your flow is tapping into energy that's not inherently yours. It's ours; it belongs to the collective.

Arranging the dispensing of your finite energy according to an "in-equals-out" approach makes sense in the context of particle-based Newtonian physics, where we thought mass was what it looked like—solid and finite. But the new science of quantum physics defies linear cause and effect; rather, "the field" organizes itself, donating mysterious and near-invisible sources of energy to those seemingly solid particles for outcomes that would have been otherwise impossible to predict. The rules change: the less you do, the less you control; the simpler and quieter you get, the *more* magically gets done; and the *greater* your sense of safety, the *more abundant* and rich your life experience.

Adopting a more quantum approach, all you need to do is get out of your own way and sign up to simply ride the wave. In this type of lifestyle, nothing is simply good or simply bad; rather, all is part of a greater design that you cannot envision from your standpoint. In this model, you are supported by a bigger web of organization. You are a part of some greater whole. And you are delivered exactly what you need, exactly when you need it. It is something you *feel*, because you are tapping into an energy flow that is universal.

Accessing this flow can be a spontaneous awakening, or it can be, as I witness daily in my clinical approach to healing, a natural outcropping of physical healing and a truce with your body. It's a way of sensing the path of your life through portals other than your eyes and ears. It's about the power of your clear mind to literally generate potential and possibility that shouldn't logically be there.

So take inventory on your mental and emotional tenants, your thoughts and your feelings. Make sure you want to renew their lease. And see what life would feel like if you sent them packing and let nature grow some breathtaking scenescape where those dingy tenements once loomed.

---

### Resetter: Ali

There is something happening to me that is taking me to places I've never imagined. I'm seeing life from an existential view instead of having the day-to-day "white-knuckling" I used to experience all the time. I see myself being plugged into the universe and am beginning to hear and feel where I'm most needed. Coincidences are happening at a daily rate, like meeting just the right person at just the right time. There is no fear for me in this—I've begun to not even be surprised when it happens because it happens so often. I listen, I observe, and I watch. I pause before I react.

This is better than any drug anyone could take—it's amazing.

---

## THE PATH TOWARD YOUR INNER INFINITY

On the path that takes you beyond your Dark Night—the one where your pure childself assumed her rightful position in your heart, in harmony with your adult consciousness, and your illusory self died—you'll find that the journey is not quite over yet. The spiritual path winds ever more into the wild unknown with tests, challenges, and revelations, serving to awaken you to all of the places where you were still asleep. It can be exhausting and feel unrelenting. This is why, for some, it can become essential to connect directly to source energy, to the divine, or to what some call the Godspace in order to feel and experientially know that everything is, in fact, perfect.

Here are some tools to aid you in connecting to the mystical within and without, so you can tap into the field of possibilities and feel the mystery, awe, and joy of life. These include (but are certainly not limited to!): silent meditation, psychedelics, White Tantric/deeper Kundalini practice and training, Qigong, Holotropic Breathwork, and dance.

### Tool #1: Psychedelics for Therapy and Mysticism

Once the emblem of a revolutionary counterculture, psychedelics are now the subject of medical research into therapeutic uses.[6] But their use also has much to tell us about mystical states that give us access to faith in a greater design. Mystical experiences are the portal to this greater perspective and are often described as being more real that "reality" as we know it, forever etched into consciousness as a life-defining shift.

*[Mystical experiences are] those peculiar states of consciousness in which the individual discovers himself to be one continuous process with God, with the Universe, with the Ground of Being, or whatever name he may use by cultural conditioning or personal preference for the ultimate and eternal reality.*

— ALAN WATTS, *PSYCHEDELICS AND RELIGIOUS EXPERIENCE*

The potential for psychedelics to bring about such states of consciousness has been known for some time. Dr. Stanislav Grof, transpersonal psychiatrist and pioneering researcher in altered states, wrote in his foreword to Albert Hoffman's 1980 book *LSD: My Problem Child* that the potential significance of LSD and other psychedelics for psychiatry is comparable to the value the microscope has for biology or the telescope for astronomy.

Today, psychedelics are entering a renaissance, and it may be because, as Michael Pollan says in *How to Change Your Mind*, "There are times in the evolution of a species when the old patterns no longer avail, and the radical, potentially innovative perceptions and behaviors that psychedelics sometimes inspire, may offer the best chance for adaptation."[7]

There's plenty of science behind the use of *entheogens* for therapy (entheogens are defined medically as a chemical substance, typically of plant origin, that is ingested to produce a nonordinary state of consciousness for religious or spiritual purposes). Studies showing beneficial effects of entheogens for depression are mounting,[8,9] with psilocybin being the most extensively studied.[10]

With response rates up to 80 percent for anxiety and depression, plants such as the psilocybin mushroom may help us be able to feel more. In fact, whereas antidepressants dampen amygdala responses to negative images, psilocybin, like compassion meditation, actually enhances these responses.[11]

Interestingly, most studies noted that there were no serious adverse effects, toxicities, or dependency when psychiatric patients were treated with entheogens. Incredibly, as of this writing, psilocybin has been licensed by the FDA for study in the treatment of drug-resistant depression.

In addition to psychedelics being studied for psychiatric diagnoses, several studies have shown that these entheogens can lead to increased mindfulness, cooperation, and pro-environmental behaviors. In one study that explored the potential of ayahuasca, an Amazonian vine used in a ceremonial brew by the same name, to increase mindfulness capacities, it was found that ayahuasca indeed reduced judgmental processing and inner reactivity, which are goals of meditation practices.[12] Another study showed that ayahuasca significantly increased divergent thinking and decreased convergent thinking, suggesting that this entheogen enhances creativity and decreases a person's sense of limitations.[13] Interestingly, people with more psychedelic experiences are more likely to construe themselves as part of nature and feel interconnectedness, leading to pro-environmental behavior.[14]

Entheogens have a capacity to foster a deep sense of connectedness to the web of life—to the natural world, to each other, to the cosmos. This connection makes it impossible to proceed with life as it is offered by the dominant paradigm, where nature is something to be managed and utilized, where production of goods and procurement of money matter, and where our bodies are thought of as machines prone to senseless malfunction. Many people describe a difference between life before even a single psychedelic experience and life after. And the "after" is characterized by a deep sense of existential arrival and ease—an experience of clarity often offered through a harrowing journey wherein the ego is shed, fractured, and left by the side of the road.

**No quick fix.** While these fast-track opportunities can offer an embodied experience of contact with the spiritual realm, they typically still entail spiritual work and commitment to integrate epiphanic realizations into daily life. In fact, this integration, the ability to hold Reality alongside reality, is why and how these agents can sometimes be destabilizing for the unprepared journeyer. For these reasons, the proper context, guidance, support, and informed consent are a vital part of the potential for healing that these experiences can offer.

My patients never take psychedelics during their tapering processes; however, they do meet with the same inner darkness and ego dissolution that can be visited through the experience of psychedelic journeys. This brink of consciousness—when traversed, embraced, and subsumed—can represent a kind of death of a former self and a rebirth into a new, expanded self-agency. The survival of this trial is highly disruptive to an illusory "normal." In fact, the cost of one's new life is their old life. And everything is subject to review, calibration, and reintegration.

A critical definitional feature of the mystical experience is a sense of unity, or the experience of becoming one with all that exists.

One would rightly imagine that this sense of unity is particularly elusive for those who have a history of violent sexual abuse, particularly incest. I have had the privilege of walking the post-taper path with my patient Sasha, who was called to explore plant medicine after tapering off 21 years of medication with a mood stabilizer, opiate, antidepressant, and two benzodiazepines. Her remarkable self-reclamation experience is pending publication, and she had this to share about an experience with plant medicine that she engaged in the year after she discontinued her medication:

> That night, I looked at so, so many dark things—things that I have long been too afraid to look at. Much of what I saw was around childhood abuse or other subsequent assaults, and I was able to see all of them without judgment. I recalled new assaults and details for the first time, but the remembering did not dismantle me as it has in the past (i.e., during talk therapy). This allowed me to look much further than I've been able to before.
>
> I quickly saw that my illnesses/remaining struggles (psoriasis, vulva pain, back pain, etc.) are all forms of self-punishment, directed by me. I didn't fully realize that I've held on to a great deal of shame and guilt, which I learned more about when seeing the things I feared most in the journey, and those things led me to turn on myself as a child—with hitting myself, etc.
>
> During the journey, I held my father and his friend's faces and forgave all of them; that came very easily. It was not quite so easy to extend that forgiveness to myself.
>
> I realized that the thing I fear the most is myself—not my father, or any outward thing, but fear of what I might do to myself, if I turn on myself.
>
> I also realized that I have held myself as a victim for some time; this was not in my awareness beforehand but seemed near impossible to get around given my past story. But I can see now how my family and I essentially co-created a story together and that is how it played out. We came to

challenge each other in a unique way during this lifetime. And the victim label is one I'm ready to shed; it no longer serves me.

It is remarkable to be able to frame up some of the darkest, most unkind memories and see them as just memories— not something I need to hold on to, or fall apart over. A part of my story, my past, that has helped get me here. I really did see it all without judgment.

At present I feel nothing but motherly love for my many abusers, which I absolutely, never, ever, ever expected would be possible. I didn't even dare to dream it.

New, glorious tracks have been laid down in this woman's life that seemingly made the impossible possible for her. But psychedelics are not the only way to break new ski tracks on fresh powder. Deep meditation practices such as silent meditation, White Tantric Kundalini Yoga, Qigong, Holotropic Breathwork, and even dance can also dissolve the construct created by our dominant beliefs for long enough to allow us to see that there *is* a curtain, let alone what's behind it.

First find yourself; then find totality. I believe that an experience of self-agency and physical healing is best to precede these portals of accelerated consciousness, that there might be a natural order of operations lest these tools overwhelm an immature mindset with energies that have no proper context to be received and worked with. Through physical healing, an alignment with the miracle of the body can afford an expanded mindset, one ready to support a deeper transformation into your most authentic self.

## Tool #2: Silent Meditation—Do Nothing

One of the most effective tools I know of to help you access the divine is *silent meditation*.

A few years ago, I began to get multiple recommendations from different sources that I needed to get quiet. Get quiet? Well, that's not hard. I love reading and writing, and thinking on my own. I do yoga and SoulCycle, and I dance, and I don't talk to anyone during those hours. That's what I thought was meant by getting quiet.

Then I understood more clearly what the challenge was: get quiet and *do nothing*. My resistance flared like a mama bear protecting her coddled babies. *No way. I don't have time for that!*

And then I forced myself. I took the plunge. I scheduled half a day, alerted my team and my family, and walked outside. No phone, no pen, no paper. Just me, my legs, and my chattering mind. I walked for three hours in silence. It felt excruciating. I almost jumped ship several times as a flood of tasks, thoughts, and even inspirations rushed in. I told myself story after story about how I needed to make this time worthwhile. I needed to get something out of it if I wasn't going to be doing something with it. Well, isn't that just productivity dressed up in a self-betterment costume?

Finally, in the last 45 minutes or so, I let go. I felt my feet moving. I used the mantra *Sat Nam*—truth is my identity—with every step. And I finally felt a bit of surrender to just being there. I touched that elusive sense that the car was going to get where it needed to go even if I wasn't slamming on the gas. I felt that maybe I didn't need to always drive. That I just needed to be aware I was in the car, check out the scenery, and enjoy the ride.

I've incorporated this kind of silent meditation into my life—initially weekly and now once a month for one to three hours. This simple behavior is responsible for a massive shift in my consciousness, giving me a sense of awe around the power of simple things to heal: food, movement, sleep, sunlight, and contact with nature.

## Shinrin-Yoku ("Forest Bathing")

The Japanese practice of Shinrin-yoku, or forest bathing, has been studied in a trial setting to quantify the known benefits, which are an improved sense of vitality and mood, and decreased anxiety and anger. A crossover trial showed that even 15 minutes of walking in the forest relative to an urban setting resulted in "lower concentrations of cortisol, lower pulse rate, lower blood pressure, greater parasympathetic nerve activity, and lower sympathetic nerve activity."[15]

Researchers theorize that breathing in volatile compounds from trees and organic decay signals our immune system, resulting in these favorable shifts. We have a long history of harmony with this ecosystem. Remember that, because your body does. In an age of 5G networks, cell towers, and ubiquitous electromagnetic pollution, it has never been more important to ground and get your feet onto the earth to literally calibrate your energy field in the way only the earth can. In fact, the clinical significance of direct contact with the earth's surface has been reviewed and researched by enlightened clinicians like Dr. Stephen Sinatra, who recommends 15 minutes a day of grounding as a wellness practice.[16]

Perhaps most importantly, I've learned that we can shift our consciousness, our psychology, and our life experience by sending ourselves meta-signals. These are big messages delivered through small behaviors. When my patients decide to follow my one-month diet and lifestyle recommendations—eat nutrient-dense foods, balance blood sugar, eliminate inflammatory foods—they are engaging in a ritual of alignment with the natural world, with honoring their organism, and with mindful engagement.

When you take hours out of your busyness to walk around aimlessly, in solitude, in nature, you are sending yourself the signal that *there is time after all.* You are walking the walk of abundance. When you act like there's time to experience beauty in nature, things begin to shift so that there actually *is* time. See what happens if you start acting like you have all the time in the world. You might just find that you do.

For a more formal practice of silent meditation, consider signing up for a Vipassana retreat.[17] *Vipassana*, which means "to see things as they really are," is one of India's most ancient techniques of meditation. Gautama Buddha rediscovered it more than 2,500 years ago and taught it as a universal remedy for universal ills.

There are no charges for Vipassana courses—not even to cover the cost of food and accommodation. All expenses are met by donations from people who, having completed a course and experienced the benefits of Vipassana, wish to give others the opportunity to also benefit.

Undertaking an intensive, silent meditation is described by many as one of the most challenging but rewarding experiences of their lives. Five to eleven days in a room full of meditators without much guidance, without pen, paper, or books, the expectation is to confront head-on all of the roadblocks that your mind and body might throw up, and to just simply be. In full disclosure, this is too ascetic a practice for me. If you are already a self-depriving, rigid go-getter, this approach to spiritual emergence may be too renunciative for you.

## Tool #3: White Tantric/Advanced Kundalini

A number of my patients and online participants go on to pursue Kundalini teacher training, now available throughout the world. This deep experience is not only for those who plan to teach, but is a self-development experience of incredible transformational potential. As a part of this training, or independent of it, White Tantric events are scheduled in various locations that present a day long intensive opportunity to experience altered states of consciousness through partner (could be a friend, lover, or stranger) meditation in a large group.[18]

Designed to break through subconscious blocks in the space of an eight-hour session, White Tantric Yoga workshops consist of between six and eight kriyas. A kriya is a meditation incorporating:

- A yoga posture (asana)
- A hand position (mudra)
- A breathing technique (pranayama)
- A mental focus and/or a mantra

Sometimes the kriyas are accompanied by music. They can vary in length up to 62 minutes, and there are breaks in between each one. The environment is peaceful, and the atmosphere is friendly, supportive, and uplifting.

## Tool #4: Wisdom Healing Qigong

Bringing them straight out of the Chinese "Medicine-less Hospital," Master Mingtong Gu has brought the radically powerful ancient self-healing protocols of Qigong to the U.S. Consisting of simple movements, visualization, and sounds, this modality has risen to the top of my list for liberating the body from stuck patterns of illness.

The outcomes from the Medicine-less Hospital in China are right up my alley, documenting an effectiveness rate in 99 percent of 200,000 cases.[19] As I was writing this chapter, I watched a YouTube of Qigong masters shrinking a three-inch bladder tumor in a patient at the Medicine-less Hospital, in real time, in less than three minutes.

Master Mingtong Gu runs a retreat center in Santa Fe, New Mexico, that has brought this ancient technology to the West, for direct training on accessing this healing field that is around us at every moment. He also teaches online, offering sound healing and a basic series called Awakening Vitality that entrains the fluid movement of energy through the body. I send anyone in need of deep redirection and connection to the healing field of energy his way, especially children and their parents.[20]

## Tool #5: Holotropic Breathwork

Holotropic Breathwork is a powerful technique for self-exploration and personal empowerment that relies on our innate capacity to move us toward wholeness. Created by transpersonal psychologists Stanislav and Cristina Grof, Holotropic Breathwork is usually done in groups, although individual sessions are also possible.[21]

The theoretical framework integrates modern consciousness research, anthropology, various depth psychologies, transpersonal psychology, Eastern spiritual practices, and mystical traditions of the world. The name *Holotropic* literally means "moving toward wholeness" (from the Greek *holos*, meaning "whole," and *trepein*, meaning "moving in the direction of something").

The process itself combines accelerated breathing with evocative music in a special setting. While lying on a mat with eyes closed, each person uses their own breath and the music in the room to enter nonordinary states of consciousness, activating the natural inner healing process of the individual's psyche. With inner healing intelligence guiding the process, the quality and content brought forth is unique to each person and for that particular time and place. While recurring themes are common, no two sessions are ever alike.

## Tool #6: Ecstatic Dance

Personally, dance is my medicine as well as my connection to the divine. When I let music move my body, I entrust that ancient creative force to clear stuck emotion and bring me to a simple place of joy. I have finally come to a place in my life where I prioritize this commitment over all others and schedule everything around dance classes that I attend six days a week. I often cry during these hours, releasing tears of stuck emotions that might otherwise stagnate and settle. I feel my soul land in my body. And after class, when I encounter an intense triggering of fear, pain, or anger, I find some alone time and turn on music I know will help me metabolize that old energy, perhaps once and for all.

Try it on your own, in a class, or in the form of "ecstatic dance," which is a nationwide phenomenon involving a climaxing playlist and free-form movement, often in a dimly lit room. It's called ecstatic dance because it can bring you there. Dance is our birthright, and as my African dance teacher, Kukuwa, explained to me, indigenous people don't learn to dance. They simply do, as their elders do, every day. She also happens to be over 60, with six-pack abs, and emanates more joy than one person can seemingly contain. She dances every day, and always has.

## CONCLUSION: THE CALL

If I have inspired you to believe that challenges—and even adversity—hold a meaning, that the body has an innate wisdom, and that the cosmos operates under the principles of an elegant design, you are ready to bend and flow with what comes. To bring curiosity to bear. And to live a life that is free of bad luck, a broken body, and emergencies.

Let me be frank: We need you. I need you. Awakening, vital, and holding the vibration of possibility. Because it is from this energy that solutions will emerge. Solutions to the big mess we've made. And solutions that cannot be drawn from the programs of the consciousness that created them. So we need to walk into the unknown, blaze new trails, and trust that the stone will appear under each foot we lift.

I believe that those who find themselves on this path are here as sentinels to anchor this process for all of humanity. You are the imaginal cells that hold the instructions for the butterfly even as the caterpillar oozes into a protoplasmic blob.

In the words of Dr. Nicholas Gonzalez:

> We are in "times of trouble" to be followed by the light of peace, the calm of hope realized, the transcendence of truth. Not now, not yet, but soon. We are in the *Suntaleia*, the Greek term for Consummation of the Ages, a time of confusion, political strife, hatred of truth, governmental oppression and the rise toward one world dictatorship. Then comes the destruction of truth's enemies, the restoration of the earth and recognition for those that gallantly stood firm for the truth and its always righteous application. So do not despair, it isn't necessary to do so, the plan is falling into place, these times are but the birth pangs of the glorious world that will follow.

I know that it may not be clear why you are destined for this hugely important role, but know that because of your awakened heart, you are now able to connect to the most vulnerable among us, to feel their pain because you have explored these depths yourself. I know that the price of admission to this awakened life is steep. It is the hardest passage you will ever traverse. It is your initiation to yourself, complete with the death of a false self built on childhood projections. Now you are ready to navigate the world from your adult consciousness, identifying your unmet needs with compassion and personal responsibility and taking care of your childself as the deepest and most tender part of what makes you strong and powerful.

And when you waver, when you feel disempowered, you'll run your checklist: Can I optimize sleep, nutrition, detox, meditation? Is there a relationship dynamic that is sucking my life force? Is it time to give myself permission to leave my job? Am I encountering emotional states related to unresolved wounds and unmet childhood needs? Am I breaking a karmic cycle that has been handed down through generations? You will no longer default to a belief that you are broken. Because you now know . . . there is not now and never was anything wrong with you.

You'll also know that what you are encountering is happening for you, not to you. You'll continue to drop your victim stories, and you'll rise to level up your healing.

And you'll always see a hand held out in the dark, reaching back to help you forward. You'll feel my hand, her hand, his hand, the hand of someone who has had the audacity to walk this path before you, leading you home . . . to yourself.

# APPENDIX A

## Peaceful Parenting

The most powerful gift you can give to your children is your own self care, and the most powerful gift they give to you is the opportunity to practice mastery of your internal emotional reactivity, the true path to peace and unconditional love.

C8 80

"I hate it here! You didn't even care about my opinion when I said I don't want to move!"

It was late when my daughter started crying, and my mind reeled as I felt sucked into what I imagined to be an emotional black hole of no return. I mounted my defense: *But you love it here! And I did involve you in the process! And do you have any idea what I've had to sacrifice to create the life you have?!* But I zipped it. I took long, deep breaths, I reached out my hand to touch her back, and I let her cry and rage, telling myself, *She's just feeling. She's just feeling.* And then, she got up, got a tissue, and hopped into bed laughing about what her nose sounded like when she blew it.

This was one of the proudest experiences of my life. That I had come to a point where I could simply let my own daughter feel her feelings without meddling, manipulating, or managing her experience required something huge on my part: it required that I feel strong enough to weather the storm inside me, and the feelings of rejection and loss of control that were seemingly induced by her emotions but that really have been living in *me* for most of my life. I showed myself, and her, that I could give her an experience of love even as we were in seeming disagreement and discord. And she showed me, and herself, that she was strong enough to share her feelings and to let that energy move through her.

## WHERE DID IT ALL START?

This simple episode was a powerful reminder to me that parenting is one of the most intense spiritual crucibles possible (seconded only by an imago-match relationship!) and that the self-authority and readiness required to show up to these beloved beings with an open heart are immense.

The challenge is particularly intense because most of us were not modeled unconditional love. At best, we were parented by "fair-weather parents" who were nice and kind or cold and sharp, depending on how our behavior suited them in the moment. At worst, we were abused, manipulated, or abandoned, left to feel like we were worthless or were some sort of an asset to be used.

And this was how we learned what love is. We learned from people who themselves were struggling, disconnected, and afraid, and who were conditioned by a culture that only knows one way to interact with powerful energies: to attempt to dominate and control them. Remember that we are several hundred years into a medical paradigm that is basically an arena for warfare on the body (antibiotics, antidepressants, anti-hypertensives). We don't care about the why; we just want the symptom to go away. So is it any surprise that our parents, and their parents, only cared about behaviors that felt good to be around? The deficiencies of this behavioral focus, without any deeper curiosity around the "why" of what a child is experiencing, is explored in the important book *Unconditional Parenting* by Alfie Kohn.

In this tour of how to disengage a "doing to" model of parenting, Kohn compassionately indicts all of the reflexive idioms we've handed down from our parents—*because I said so, this is a privilege, not a right, there's no dessert until you . . .* —and he uses the example of the forced apology to illustrate the bankruptcy of the behavioral model. He states that when we force a child to apologize to another, we are interested only in the behavior conformity, not in their actually feeling apologetic—in effect, stripping the behavior of its deeper moral meaning and rendering it a lie.

In this way, we set up a paradigm where our children are sharing because we say, "Good job sharing, Billy!" and not because it feels good to give; they are getting good grades in school not because it feels good to learn; and they are beginning the process of hiding, suppressing, and otherwise denying the aspects of themselves that seem to garner love withdrawal and punishment.

The incentives for ethical behavior get externalized onto a grid of goodness and badness according to the meritocracy and value system that parents establish. Lost is the inner compass, the inner sense of one's needs, including around nourishing themselves and expressing their emotions. And ultimately we can be left having followed all the rules, played nice, and still feeling fundamentally unfulfilled, unwelcome, unliked, and even unloved on a soul level.

## DON'T PUNISH, DON'T REWARD

Kohn takes the provocative position that any parental behavior that gives children a feeling of less access to love, including time-outs, results in an internal distortion in the child. He goes so far as to say, "These responses—calculating the risks, figuring out how not to get caught, lying to protect oneself—make sense from the child's perspective. They're perfectly rational. What they're not is moral, and that's because punishment—all punishment, by its very nature—impedes moral thinking."[1]

He then takes rewards and praise off of the table, stating, "The more people are rewarded for something, the more likely they are to lose interest in whatever they had to do to get the reward."[2]

As I read this, I reflected on my résumé of conventionally laudable achievements and how none of them felt the way one might have thought they would. In fact, I don't remember feeling genuine deep pride the way I did that night with my daughter when I graduated MIT or medical school, fellowship, published my first paper, or had a *New York Times* bestseller. And I'm not the only one. Achievement-motivated behavior is an adult compensation for the love we don't believe would otherwise be there, but it doesn't feel like real love. It feels like an endless black hole.

And that is the feeling we give our children when we make them feel that who they are, what they are feeling, and how they've chosen to behave closes our heart to them. This kind of rejection feels like an existential threat to a child who is navigating this wild world, and it conditions them to develop what Kohn calls "contingent self-esteem."

Know anyone who only feels good about themselves when they get positive feedback? How many of us could tap into a reservoir of self-love, even when there's no evidence of love coming from anywhere in our life? That's what superficial and fleeting self-esteem feels like.

This is what I seek to untangle in myself, and in my patients who have been medicated because of a deeply held belief that what they are feeling is wrong, and that they are in the end wrong, broken, and unlovable—unless they are good patients who take their pills and get back to the regularly scheduled program.

Kohn writes, "It makes perfect sense, then, that the most striking long-term effect of love withdrawal is fear. Even as young adults, people who were treated that way by their parents are still likely to be unusually anxious. They may be afraid to show anger. They tend to display a significant fear of failure. And their adult relationships may be warped by a need to avoid attachment—perhaps because they live in dread of being abandoned all over again."[3]

Check, check, and check.

So how do we break the cycle? Motherhood has given me an opportunity to say, the buck stops here, and then to commit to consciousness in every moment of my waking life. And when I lapse, commit again. This commitment has required that I turn away from my productivity addiction and achievement orientation and toward the simple aspects of life that I thought were somehow optional. This commitment has required me to s-l-o-w down and learn how to just be in my day, in my life, in a room with my daughters with no plan.

And it has required a deep commitment to a personal meditation practice, self-care, and work with my family of origin so I could grow strong enough to stay present and in control during my internal emotional storms when my daughters inevitably trip my wires. So I can tell myself, *Kelly, you can handle this . . . these are feelings happening, and there's nothing to do but let them happen.*

This parenting-induced growth seems universally available to us if we choose to say yes to it. One Resetter wrote:

> My four-year-old daughter, Sara, took apart a handmade mobile I had made for her when she was a babe, complete with a red cardinal centerpiece. She was in a full-on tantrum, nothing made sense. She was overtired and lay screaming as I tried to soothe her baby brother to sleep.
>
> I felt the fire blaze inside me. But . . . I finally kept my cool and turned inward although my skin turned hot. I felt my triggers being pulled and instead of reacting out of habit, I gently released the grip. I acknowledged my pain, felt it, and let it go. Poof.
>
> She eventually ended up a puddle on my lap, as I began to rock her to sleep. I whispered, "You are whole, you are okay, you are complete." She nodded as if she already knew and peacefully drifted away, like a ship safely making it to its shore.
>
> My whole being and perspective changed at that moment. My body tingled. I realized . . . I wasn't just saying that to my daughter, I was saying it to myself—to my past, to my present, and to my future self.

And I'm saying it to each of you. . . . Children can be our greatest teachers and we, we are our greatest healers.

This is the hardest and most rewarding work I've ever done, and I invite you to consider this commitment for yourself and for your children. Because we know, in our hearts, that our children are not opponents, and that there has to be more to parenting than domination and control.

As Kohn writes, "It's harder to make sure children feel loved unconditionally than it is to just love them," and I would say this goes for all relationships.[4] If you say you love someone but they don't feel it, it may be because you have given them the experience of being conditionally received, and that resentment and guardedness lie between you under the *I heart you* birthday cards.

So how do we give our children a feeling of our openheartedness at all times? This openheartedness is the defining feature of divine connection, so naturally, it will help to orient toward your children as expressions of the divine. As fundamentally already whole and perfect, no matter what. If this feels tough to embrace, it's probably because you have been brainwashed by our child-resenting culture to assume that children are fundamentally bad and have ill intent that needs to be controlled and managed. Sounds something like our adult perceptions around laws, rules, and health. Rather than seeing that we have agreed on conditions that give rise to struggle and suffering, we would prefer to see our conditions as just and those expressing the wrongness of those conditions as the problem.

Natalie Christensen of the Center for Emotional Education[5] has the following recommendations for meeting the inevitable challenges that parenting brings:

1.  **Notice:** Notice when your child is shifting into an uncomfortable emotional brain state, losing the ability to function cognitively, losing impulse control, losing the ability to empathize, losing optimism, motivation, and/or composure. Notice this shift, and also notice how it feels to you. Often the first clue to what your child is experiencing is how you are feeling about it. If you feel powerless, they likely are too. If you feel angry, that's a good guess for your child as well. Look for it in your body. And then notice your child's body. Where/how is it showing up?

2.  **Name.** Help your child process through naming their feelings. Neuro-emotional co-processing in this manner is how our brains are designed for us to support each other in times of trauma: we network our suffering so it doesn't overwhelm any one system. With our children, and over time, neuro-emotional co-processing trains their brains to be better at managing feelings and intense situations without "melting down."

3.  **Touch.** Use physiological cues to tell your child's nervous system that they are safe enough to let their emotions be expressed. If your child has sunk into a "fight-flight-freeze-appease" mode—in their lower brain and para- and sympathetic nervous systems—they may not readily welcome physical contact but might be okay with proximity. In this state, you approach as you would in attempting to pet a feral cat: slowly, gently, reassuringly, sometimes barely moving but staying near, communicating with your body, countenance, and energy that you are safe and trustworthy. You might only be allowed to be in the same room at first, then maybe on the same piece of furniture, then possibly a finger on a toe, then hopefully full hugs, or some variation on this theme.

4.  **Wait/repeat.** As you may have gleaned from #3, the real work here is waiting. It takes time for all the tears to come out, for all the naming words to be said, for all the hugs to be had, and for physiology to catch up with brain chemistry. Consider your time to be a front-end investment, because if you don't put in that time, your child's emotion just snowballs. Sooner or later, you have to put in the time to address it anyway. So best to wait in these moments with your upset child, hearing them out, connecting over this feeling and all the ones that come after, investing your time in the relationship and in brain function.

For support and cultivation of this ethos in your family, my daughter and I wrote an illustrated children's book called *A Time for Rain* about the meaning and deep purpose of difficult feelings. Let's start a new kind of curriculum: one that honors emotions as a child's primary entitlement.

# APPENDIX B

## Natural Medicine Toolkit

Here are some of the "always have at home" essentials I recommend to help you support your body's recalibration around stressors, conflicts, and detox. While the research supports the "antimicrobial" effects of these compounds and foods, the truth is that they speak to the body in ways we are only beginning to understand and may never be able to quantify.

### HERBS, SUPPLEMENTS, AND OTHER SUPPORTS

**Botanical herbs:** For centuries, botanical herbs have been used as antibiotics. Since there are countless herbal remedies for various types of infections[1,2,3] I'll just list a few common herbs that have been validated by modern research. For example, the herb *Inula helenium*, also called *elecampane*, was shown to be 100 percent effective against 200 isolates of *Staphylococcus aureus* (commonly known as "staph infection").[4] Similarly, a study that evaluated *Alpinia galanga*, a plant in the ginger family that has been traditionally used in Asian countries, found that this herb was effective against *Salmonella typhi* and *E. coli*, as well as against other drug-resistant bacterial strains.[5] Extract from *Nigella sativa*, a flowering plant native to South Asia, kills MRSA, methicillin-resistant *Staphylococcus aureus*,[6] while cinnamon and oregano are potent selective antibiotics against many drug-resistant species.[7] Similarly, easy-to-find spices like cumin[8] and rosemary[9] are powerful antimicrobials, as are child-friendly options like elderberry.[10,11] Many high-quality herbal combination products combine evidence-based herbs such as oregano,[12,13] echinacea,[14,15,16] and goldenseal[17,18,19] into an effective immune support formula.

**Mushrooms:** According to preeminent mycologist Paul Stamets, mushrooms can save the world,[20] and medicinal mushrooms have a long history in the healing practices of many cultures, so it is no surprise that medical literature supports their robust effect on your immune system.[21]

Paul's recently published research[22] explores another fundamental way in which fungi communicate with humanity: through our digestive systems. Mushrooms are prebiotic, boosting the microbiome's beneficial bacteria, such as *acidophilus* and *bifidobacterium*, improving digestion and overall health.[23]

AHCC (*active hexose correlated compound*) from shitake mushrooms is classified as a functional food made from hybridized mycelia of shiitake (and sometimes other mushrooms); it contains both alpha- and beta-glucan polysaccharides, well-known modulators of host immunity. Culinary shiitake mushrooms, eaten daily, have been found to boost quantifiable factors related to immunity, such as populations of natural killer T cells.[24]

Most immune support blends include several researched mushrooms, and Paul Stamet's preparation includes the following: royal sun blazei, cordyceps, enokitake, amadou, agarikon, artist's conk, reishi, Oregon polypore, maitake, lion's mane, chaga, shiitake, mesima, birch polypore, pearl oyster, split gill polypore, and turkey tail.

**Colloidal silver:** Also called *silver nanoparticles*, colloidal silver has been used for over 2,000 years to resolve bacterial infections.[25] As such, silver is commonly used in intravenous catheters, dental fillings, wound dressings, and bone implants.[26]

Though the exact antimicrobial mechanisms are still debated, colloidal silver is thought to damage the cell membranes of opportunistic bacteria. Depending on the surface charge of the silver nanoparticles and the type of bacteria, bacteria can be killed by the formation of free radicals, accumulation of nanoparticles in bacterial cell walls, or depletion of cell membrane components.[27] Colloidal silver is effective both as a topical treatment for skin infections like MRSA[28] and as an oral "antibiotic."[29]

**Manuka honey:** Raw manuka honey is one of the tastiest ways to stay healthy. This honey comes from bees in New Zealand that pollinate the manuka bush, and it has been used for thousands of years by various cultures to promote wellness. This high-antioxidant golden honey is a popular ingredient in high-end skin care products, as it is broadly anti-inflammatory and antimicrobial.[30] Eaten, manuka honey can cure antibiotic-resistant *C. difficile* infection,[31,32] strep throat,[33,34] urinary tract infections,[35] and MRSA, an infection caused by a type of staph bacteria that's become resistant to many of the antibiotics used to treat ordinary staph infections.[36] A bonus of eating honey is that it can include propolis, a mixture of bee saliva and wax known as "bee glue," which contains over 300 therapeutic compounds that fight cancer,[37,38] as well as potentially opportunistic bacteria.[39,40]

**Thymus glandular:** Originating from ancestral eating practices that involved the consumption of whole animals, glandular capsules are special preparations of glands and organs such as thyroid, spleen, liver, thymus, and thyroid. Dr. Gonzalez used glandulars as a foundational support in his protocol, including the immune-supportive gland, the thymus, which can be taken as three capsules three to four times a day when needed.

**N-acetyl cysteine (NAC):** From the amino acid L-cysteine, NAC is used by the liver to form glutathione, the body's primary antioxidant. NAC is a great choice as a mucolytic to loosen mucous when your body may need help expelling what's rattling around from a productive cough. Dosage is up to 1gm 2 to 3 times a day between meals. Side benefits include improvements in liver and brain inflammation.[41,42]

**Bentonite clay:** Bentonite, also known as *montmorillonite*, is composed of aged volcanic ash and is one of the most effective and powerful healing clays. The name comes from the largest known deposit of bentonite clay, located in Fort Benton, Wyoming.

Bentonite clay is unique in its ability to produce an electrical charge upon contact with fluid, enabling it to absorb and remove toxins, heavy metals, impurities, and chemicals. Bentonite clay is a common ingredient in detox and cleansing products and can be used externally as a clay poultice or mud pack, in the bath, and in skin care protocols. It has a very fine, velveteen feel and is odorless and non-staining. A good-quality bentonite is sourced as a liquid. For internal cleansing, try drinking 1 tablespoon of liquid bentonite in a cup of water most days. For significant diarrhea or stomach upset, drink 1/3 cup of liquid three times in one day.

**Vitamins D$_3$ and A:** Traditional cultures prioritized access to nutrient- and fat-rich foods, such as organ meats, fish eggs, and raw dairy that support the appropriate expression of programmable genes. These foods are rich in fat-soluble vitamins, D$_3$, A, and K$_2$, which, we are learning, appear to act in concert to support immune health and cellular signaling.

Vitamin D deficiencies are driven by glyphosate-induced impairment of synthesis in our livers, in addition to indoor lifestyles. Inspired by author and presenter Dr. Alex Vasquez's "inflammology" approach,[43] the use of the fat-soluble vitamins D$_3$ and pre-formed A at high doses for a period of four days can help restore immune-inflammatory resources and correct deficiencies that can drive anything from pain to patterns of symptoms referred to as viral infections. Dose 50,000 IU/day for one day followed by 10,000 IU/day for four days along with vitamin A 50,000 IU/day for five days.

**Vitamin C and zinc:** Studied formally for malaria, pneumonia, diarrheal infections, and more, this combination contributes to the innate immune system's capacity to self-fortify.[44,45,46]

Vitamin C, according to Dr. Suzanne Humphries,[47] who has experience treating pertussis and other seeming infections with this approach in the sodium ascorbate form, in dosages of 1g every three hours, as well as zinc picolinate 10-30mg daily for the duration of illness.

**Homeopathics: *oscillococcinum* and *arnica*.** Homeopathy is my go-to approach for any and all bodily imbalances because it has the capacity to address the energetic layers of an illness manifesting in the physical realm. While I am certified in clinical homeopathy, I highly recommend having a classical homeopath in your provider stable because of the nuance required to select constitutional remedies. That said, two easily acquired remedies include a "flu" staple, called *oscillococcinum*, and an injury staple that also comes in an ointment for swelling and bruising, called *arnica*.

**Ayurveda staples: neti pot, oil pulling, and tongue scraping.** For cleansing and detox when experiencing allergies, use a neti pot to flush your sinuses with salt water, at the first sign of congestion or even daily. Tongue scraping and oil pulling (I use coconut oil) for 3 to 20 minutes are game-changing practices for your oral microbiome.

**Healing tea:** Crush two cloves of garlic, add honey to taste (about a teaspoon to start), approximately 2 teaspoons (or one thumb's worth) minced ginger, a sprinkle of cayenne pepper, and hot filtered water. Drink three to four times when in need of support.

## Bonus Recipe: Chicken Stock

Make a pot of this weekly.

1 large onion, coarsely chopped

2 large carrots, chopped

3 celery stalks, chopped

1 (5- to 8-pound) organic pastured chicken, rinsed

2 to 4 tablespoons apple cider vinegar (½ tablespoon per quart of water)

Unprocessed sea salt and freshly ground black pepper

1 bunch (or 10 sprigs) cilantro or parsley, chopped

½ pound chicken livers (optional; when they're finely chopped, you won't taste them and they provide lots of nutrients)

Combine all the ingredients in a large stainless-steel stockpot and add cold filtered water to cover. Bring to a boil, then reduce the heat to very low, cover, and simmer for about 3 hours. A pressure cooker will cut the time in half. After the chicken is cooked, the meat can be separated from the bone and used in a shredded chicken dish by just sautéing the shredded chicken in olive oil and adding salt and lemon.

## NATURAL MEDICINE URINARY TRACT INFECTION (UTI) KIT

Urinary tract infection (UTI) is one of the most common reasons for antibiotic treatment, and it is very simple to optimize urinary and bladder imbalances. In addition to increasing your filtered water intake, consider these supports:

- **D-mannose** can support the bladder wall and has been demonstrated to be more effective than an antibiotic for UTI prevention.[48] For acute treatment take 1gm three to five times a day.

- **Vitamin C**, even in small doses, can also be used preventatively, including in pregnancy.[49]

- **Apple cider vinegar**, 1 tablespoon three times a day, can also help support the microbiome of the bladder.[50]

- **Oregano oil** is a powerful antibiotic alternative, also available in higher-dose supplement form in doses around 200mg, three times a day.[51]

- **Cantharis 30C** is a homeopathic remedy for urinary burning; take three to five pellets once and monitor for effect. Dose every few hours up to three times before assessing efficacy.[52]

- **Fists of Anger Meditation**. Thought by Louise Hay to represent anger, particularly around past issues in relationships, UTIs can be helped by this three-minute meditation.[53]
  - **Mudra:** Touch each thumb to the base of the Mercury (pinky) fingers. Close the rest of the fingers over the thumbs to form fists. Raising the arms, begin a backstroke type movement over the head, alternating each side (right/left) as you swing up, over, and back around again.

- **Breath:** Through an O-shaped mouth, begin strong, rhythmic inhale/exhale in sync with arm movements.

- **Position:** Sit on your knees or cross-legged, with light jalandhar bandh (chin tucked in with back of head pulled up as if by a string). Eyes are closed.

- **Intentionally** think about anything and everything that makes you angry. Continue this laser focus on bringing up the anger throughout the meditation, increasing the movement and breath.

- **To End:** Interlock the fingers, stretch the arms up overhead, palms facing up, and inhale deeply through the O mouth. Picture yourself surrounded in white, healing light and exhale out the O mouth. Repeat three times.

- **Time:** 3 minutes.

## HEALING MEDITATIONS/EXERCISES

Here are three simple yogic practices you can incorporate into your natural medicine tool kit for help with headache, general immunity, and self-healing.

### For headaches[54]

- Lie flat on your back. Stretch your arms out on the floor above your head. Spread your legs wide apart.

- Inhale and sit up, stretching forward to touch your hands to the floor between your legs. Exhale back down onto your back.

- Continue 26 times. (Caution: if you have back problems, consult your doctor before trying this exercise.)

### For general immunity[55]

1. Sit in Easy Pose (on the floor, with legs crossed) with your chin in and your chest out.

2. Stick your tongue all the way out and keep it out as you rapidly breathe in and out through your mouth. This is called Dog Breath. Continue this panting diaphragmatic breath for 3 to 5 minutes.

3. To finish, inhale and hold your breath for 15 seconds and press the tongue against the upper palate. Exhale. Repeat this sequence two more times.

## For self-healing[56]

Known as the Ultimate Healing Tool, this meditation has been used by Kundalini Yoga practitioners for the last four and a half decades. Try it when you want to send healing energy to a loved one or need healing yourself.

1. **Posture:** Sit in Easy Pose (on the floor, with legs crossed) or in a chair with feet planted firmly on the ground, with the spine straight and a light neck lock applied (chin pulled back slightly).

2. **Mudra:** The mudra (hand position) is most important. The elbows are bent down by the sides and are tucked comfortably but firmly against the ribs. The forearms are almost perpendicular to the floor, with the hands extended out at a 45-degree angle from the center of the body. Most importantly, the palms are perfectly flat, facing up, hands bent back at the wrists. You should feel a pull in the lowest part of your forearm as you almost hyperextend your wrist to make the palms flat. (This tends to be the most challenging part of the meditation, so it is important not to let the hands relax out of the position.) The fingers are kept side by side, except that the thumb is spread from the other four fingers.

3. **Eyes:** Eyes are closed.

4. **Mantra:** This mantra consists of eight basic sounds: Ra Ma Da Sa, Sa Say So Hung. They translate as follows:

Ra—Sun

Ma—Moon

Daa—Earth

Saa—Impersonal Infinity

Saa Say—Totality of Infinity

So—Personal sense of merger and identity

Hung—The infinite, vibrating and real

This mantra taps into the energies of the sun, moon, earth, and the Infinite Spirit to bring deep healing. It is important to pull the navel point powerfully on the first *Sa* and on *Hung*. The word *Hung* is not long and drawn out; rather, it is clipped off forcefully as you pull in the navel. Chant one complete cycle of the entire mantra with each breath. Then deeply inhale and repeat. Remember to move the mouth precisely with each sound. Try to feel the resonance in the mouth and in the sinus area.

5. **Mental focus:** You can choose to mentally visualize the person or persons you are wanting to heal as you send this energy to them for their well-being.

6. **Time:** Continue chanting for 11 to 31 minutes (based on yogic time intervals for energetic shifts).

7. **To end:** To end the meditation, inhale deeply and hold the breath as you offer a healing prayer. Visualize the person you wish to heal as being totally healthy, radiant, and strong. See the person completely engulfed in a healing white light and completely healed. Then exhale and inhale deeply again, hold the breath, and offer the same prayer again. Exhale.

To complete, inhale deeply, stretch your arms up high, and vigorously shake out your hands and fingers for several seconds. Keep the arms up and hands shaking as you exhale. Repeat two more times and relax.

# APPENDIX C

## Sample Meal Plan

### Paleo Pancakes

*Prep time: 10 minutes*
*Serves: 1*

½ cup cooked sweet potato or winter squash (such as butternut, acorn, or kabocha) or 1 banana

3 large pastured eggs

2 tablespoons hemp seeds, flax seeds, or nut butter

Virgin coconut oil

Combine all the ingredients except coconut oil in a blender and blend until smooth.

Heat coconut oil in a frying pan over medium heat. Spoon the batter into the pan in silver-dollar-size dollops. They cook quickly!

 cs 8o

## Cauliflower Carrot Soup

*Prep time: 35 minutes*
*Cook time: 45 minutes*
*Serves: 4*

2 tablespoons extra virgin olive oil

1 medium onion, chopped

2 cloves garlic, chopped

½ small head cauliflower (about 1lb.), cut into florets

2 carrots, peeled and chopped

1 quart vegetable broth

2 tablespoons parsley, chopped

1 tablespoon chives, chopped

1 teaspoon rosemary, chopped

1 teaspoon fresh dill, chopped

1 teaspoon celery salt

½ teaspoon salt

1 ½ cup coconut milk

Heat the oil in a 2-quart saucepot over medium heat for 1–2 minutes, or until hot.

Sauté the onions over medium heat for 3 minutes, or until they are limp and just starting to brown.

Add the garlic, cauliflower, and carrots and sauté for 5 minutes.

Add the remaining ingredients, stir well to combine, and bring the soup to a boil over medium-high heat. Lower to medium heat and simmer for 35 minutes.

Pour the soup into a blender container. Cover the container and remove the center cup from the cover. Place a clean, folded kitchen towel over the blender cover and press down with your hand. Purée the soup until smooth.

Serve immediately and refrigerate leftovers.

Cook's Note: An immersion blender is the ideal cooking tool for puréeing hot soup right in the sauce pot. If you don't have an immersion blender, you can pour the hot soup into a food processor or blender.

CB 80

# Curry Chicken

*Prep time: 20 minutes*
*Cook time: 40 minutes*
*Serves: 4*

2 tablespoons coconut oil or ghee

1 ½ pounds chicken thighs, boneless and skinless, cut into 1-inch pieces

1 medium onion, cut into large chunks

2 zucchini, thickly sliced

1 tablespoon curry powder

½ teaspoon paprika

3 cloves garlic, minced

1 teaspoon unprocessed sea salt

14 ounces unsweetened organic coconut milk

1 cup grape tomatoes

¼ cup cilantro, chopped, for garnish

In a stockpot, heat the oil or ghee to medium-high heat, then add the chicken and cook until pieces are browned on both sides, 8 to 10 minutes. Remove the chicken from the pot and set aside, leaving the remaining oil in the pot.

Add the onion and zucchini to the pot and sauté until lightly browned, about 5 minutes. Add the curry powder, paprika, garlic, and salt and sauté for half a minute.

Place the chicken pieces back in the pot and add coconut milk. Bring to a boil, then reduce heat to a simmer and cover.

Cook until chicken is tender, approximately 30 minutes. Add the tomatoes in the final 5 minutes of cooking.

Garnish with cilantro and serve.

C3 80

## Classic Pot Roast with Root Vegetables

*Prep time: 15 minutes*
*Serves: 8 to 10*

3 to 3 ½ pounds beef chuck roast

Coarse salt

1 tablespoon olive oil

2 onions, chopped

3 cloves garlic, smashed, peeled, and chopped

3 cups flavored stock (can be meat or vegetable)

3 tablespoons apple cider vinegar

Several sprigs fresh thyme

1 bay leaf

Ground black pepper

4 carrots, chopped into large pieces (leave skins on if organic)

2 small or 1 large sweet potatoes or parsnips, quartered (leave skins on if organic)

Preheat oven to 350°F.

Season the chuck roast with coarse salt. Heat a large (approximately 5-quart) Dutch oven over medium-high heat. Add the olive oil. Sear the roast on both sides in the hot Dutch oven for 5 to 6 minutes per side, then remove and set aside.

Reduce the heat to medium. Add the chopped onions and cook until softened (about 5 to 8 minutes). Add the garlic; stir and cook for 1 minute.

Place the roast back in the Dutch oven and then add the stock, vinegar, thyme, bay leaf, and black pepper. Stir and bring to a simmer.

Cover the dish and place it in the preheated oven. Cook for 2 hours.

Remove dish from the oven and add the carrots and sweet potatoes or parsnips. Place it back in the oven for another 30 minutes.

Either slice or shred the beef to serve. Use the juices in the pot as a jus or as flavored stock for the next time you make this delicious classic!

ᘓ ᘔ

## Honey Nut Bars

*Prep time: 15 minutes*
*Bake time: 20 minutes*
*Serves: 12*

1 cup cashews

½ cup almonds

½ cup pecans

½ cup unsweetened shredded coconut

½ cup cacao nibs

1 teaspoon pure vanilla extract

½ teaspoon sea salt

9 tablespoons raw honey

Preheat oven to 350°F and line an 8 x 8-inch baking pan with parchment paper.

Roughly chop the nuts into approximately ¼-inch pieces. Combine nuts with remaining ingredients, except honey, in a large bowl and stir. Add honey and mix until ingredients are evenly coated.

Spread the mixture in the pan, pressing down to pack it in and reach all the edges and corners.

Bake for 20 minutes. Cool completely on a wire rack, then cut into 12 squares.

CB&O

# ENDNOTES

## Chapter 1: Canaries in the Coal Mine

1. Substance Abuse and Mental Health Services Administration, "Key Substance Use and Mental Health Indicators in the United States: Results from the 2016 National Survey on Drug Use and Health," https://www.samhsa.gov/data/sites/default/files/NSDUH-FFR1-2016/NSDUH-FFR1-2016.pdf.

2. Graham Hancock, "The War on Consciousness—Banned TED Talk," September 30, 2013. https://www.youtube.com/watch?v=X_hShqKn5cg.

3. Charles Eisenstein, "Psychedelics and Systems Change," *MAPS Bulletin* 26, no. 1, Spring 2016 (April 19, 2016).

4. Terence McKenna, "A Message to Artists from Terence McKenna [1990]," YouTube, https://www.youtube.com/watch?v=z5wrcMiT2jM.

5. P. Jedlicka, "Revisiting the Quantum Brain Hypothesis: Toward Quantum Neuro(Biology)?", *Frontiers in Molecular Neuroscience* 10 (November 7, 2017): 366, https://www.ncbi.nlm.nih.gov/pubmed/29163041.

6. Alan Watts, *Does It Matter? Essays on Man's Relation to Materiality* (Novato, CA: New World Library, 2007).

7. Candace Pert, *Molecules of Emotion: The Science Behind Mind-Body Medicine* (New York: Simon and Schuster, 2010).

8. Pert, *Molecules of Emotion.*

9. M. Maes, "Depression Is an Inflammatory Disease, but Cell-Mediated Immune Activation Is the Key Component of Depression," *Progress in Neuro-Psychopharmacology and Biological Psychiatry* 35, no. 3 (April 29, 2011): 664–75. doi: 10.1016/j.pnpbp.2010.06.014.

10. F. Dickerson et al., "Immune Alterations in Acute Bipolar Depression," *Acta Psychiatrica Scandinavica* 132, no. 3 (September 2015): 204–10. doi: 10.1111/acps.12451.

11. Bai Ya-Mei et al., "Comparison of Inflammatory Cytokine Levels among Type I/Type II and Manic/Hypomanic/Euthymic/Depressive States of Bipolar Disorder," *Journal of Affective Disorders* Vol. 166 (September 2014), 187–92. doi: 10.1016/j.jad.2014.05.009.

12. Z. Taylor and K. Brogan, "Anxiety: Inflammatory Origins and Natural Treatments," *Price-Pottenger Journal* 38, no. 3 (October 16, 2014): 13–19.

13. Chadi A. Calarge, Sridevi Devaraj, and Robert J. Shulman, "Gut Permeability and Depressive Symptom Severity in Unmedicated Adolescents," *Journal of Affective Disorders* 246, no. 1 (March 1, 2019): 586–94. https://doi.org/10.1016/j.jad.2018.12.077.

14. S. Bengmark, "Gut Microbiota, Immune Development and Function," *Pharmacological Research* 69, Issue 1 (March 2013): 87–113.

15. B. C. Broom et al., "Symbolic Diseases and 'Mindbody' Co-emergence. A Challenge for Psychoneuroimmunology," *Explore* 8, Issue 1 (January–February 2012): 16–25. doi: 10.1016/j.explore.2011.10.005.

## Chapter 2: The Pill Problem

1. Presented to Parliament on October 7, the biennial report from Belgium's Federal Commission on the Control and Evaluation of Euthanasia confirms that 124 of the 3,950 euthanasia cases in Belgium involved persons diagnosed with a "mental and behavioral disorder" from 2014 to 2015. Lethal injections were administered, upon the request of 5 non-terminally ill people with schizophrenia, 5 with autism, 8 with bipolar disorder, 29 with dementia, and 39 with depression, according to the report. Belgium legalized euthanasia in 2002 for patient suffering "unbearably" from terminal or non-terminal conditions that are considered "untreatable." Accordingly, requests may be fulfilled within one month.

2. U.S. Department of Health and Human Services, Agency for Healthcare Research and Quality, Medical Expenditure Panel Survey through 2016,https://meps .ahrq.gov/mepsweb/data_stats/download_data_files_results. jsp?cboDataYear= All&cboDataTypeY=2%2CHousehold+Event+File&buttonYearandDataType= Search&cboPufNumber=All&SearchTitle=Prescribed+Medicines.

3. R. Mojtabai R and M. Olfson, "National Trends in Long-Term Use of Antidepressant Medications: Results from the U.S. National Health and Nutrition Examination Survey." *Journal of Clinical Psychiatry* 75, no. 2 (February 2014): 169–77. doi: 10.4088/JCP.13m08443.

4. CDC National Center for Health Statistics, National Health and Nutrition Examination Survey, updated 1/20/2019, https://www.cdc.gov/nchs/nhanes /index.htm.

5. World Health Organization, "America's State of Mind Report," 2011. The research reviewed prescription drug claims of over two million Americans to assess the use of antidepressants, antipsychotics, attention deficit hyperactivity disorder drugs and anti-anxiety treatments between 2001 and 2010.

6. According to a report presented in 2014 by the Centers for Disease Control and Prevention, 2014, and Alan Schwartz, "Thousands of Toddlers Are Medicated for A.D.H.D, Report Finds, Raising Worries," *New York Times*, May 16, 2014, https:// www.nytimes.com/2014/05/17/us/among-experts-scrutiny-of-attention-disorder-diagnoses-in-2-and-3-year-olds.html?_r=0, more than 10,000 American toddlers two or three years old are being medicated for attention deficit hyperactivity disorder (ADHD) outside established pediatric guidelines.

7. Carmen Moreno et al., "National Trends in the Outpatient Diagnosis and Treatment of Bipolar Disorder in Youth." *Archives of General Psychiatry* 64, no. 9 (September 2007): 1032–39. https://www.ncbi.nlm.nih.gov/pubmed/17768268.

8. Erick H. Turner et al., "Selective Publication of Antidepressant Trials and Its Influence on Apparent Efficacy," *New England Journal of Medicine* 358 (January 17, 2008): 252–60. doi: 10.1056/NEJMsa065779.

9. Leon Eisenberg, "Treating Depression and Anxiety in the Primary Care Setting," *Health Affairs* 11, no. 3 (Fall 1992). doi: 10.1056/NEJM199204163261610.

10. Yoichiro Takayanagi et al., "Antidepressant Use and Lifetime History of Mental Disorders in a Community Sample: Results from the Baltimore Epidemiologic Catchment Area Study," *Journal of Clinical Psychiatry* 76, no. 1 (January 2015): 40–44. doi: 10.4088/JCP.13m08824.

11. Targum, S. D., "Identification and Treatment of Antidepressant Tachyphylaxis," *Innovations in Clinical Neuroscience* 11, no. 3–4 (March 2014): 24–8.

12. R. S. El-Mallakh et al., "Tardive Dysphoria: The Role of Long Term Antidepressant Use in Inducing Chronic Depression," *Medical Hypotheses* 76, no. 6 (June 2011): 769–73.

13. Peter Breggin and David Cohen, *Your Drug May Be Your Problem: How and Why to Stop Taking Psychiatric Medications* (New York: Da Capo, 1999).

14. Irving Kirsch et al., "Do Outcomes of Clinical Trials Resemble Those 'Real World' Patients? A Reanalysis of the STAR*D Antidepressant Data Set," *Psychology of Consciousness: Theory, Research, and Practice* 5, no. 4 (December 2018): 339–45. doi: 10.1037/cns0000164.

15. Allan M. Leventhal and David O. Antonuccio, "On Chemical Imbalances, Antidepressants, and the Diagnosis of Depression," *Ethical Human Psychology and Psychiatry* 11, no. 3 (December 2009): 199–214. doi: 10.1891/1559-4343 .11.3.199.

16. Irving Kirsch and Guy Sapirstein, "Listening to Prozac but Hearing Placebo: A Meta-Analysis of Antidepressant Medication," *Prevention and Treatment* 1, no. 2, Article ID 2a (June 1998). doi: 10.1037/1522-3736.1.1.12a.

17. Irving Kirsch et al., " Initial Severity and Antidepressant Benefits: A Meta-Analysis of Data Submitted to the Food and Drug Administration," *PLoS Medicine* 5, e45 (February 26, 2008). doi: 10.1371/journal.pmed.0050045.

18. J. Moncrieff, S. Wessely, and R. Hardy, "Meta-Analysis of Trials Comparing Antidepressants with Active Placebos," *British Journal of Psychiatry* 172, no. 3 (March 1998): 227–31.

19. Alia J. Crum and Ellen J. Langer, "Mind-Set Matters: Exercise and the Placebo Effect," *Psychological Science* 18, no. 2 (February 2007): 165–71.

20. H. L. Bennett, D. R. Benson, and D. A. Kuiken, "Preoperative Instructions for Decreased Bleeding during Spine Surgery," *Anesthesiology* 65 (1986): A245.

21. Bruce Lipton, "The Biology of Belief," full lecture, 12/21/2014, https://www .youtube.com/watch?v=82ShSNuru6c.

22. M. Peciña et al., "Association Between Placebo-Activated Neural Systems and Antidepressant Responses: Neurochemistry of Placebo Effects in Major Depression," *JAMA Psychiatry* 72, no. 11 (November 2015): 1087–94. doi: 10.1001 /jamapsychiatry.2015.1335.

23. Ted J. Kaptchuk and Franklin G. Miller, "Placebo Effects in Medicine," *New England Journal of Medicine* 373, no. 1 (July 2, 2015): 8–9. doi: 10.1056 /NEJMp1504023.

24. His wisdom, resources, and evidence-based conclusions are generously offered here: https://www.madinamerica.com/anatomy-of-an-epidemic/. And this is the case for every single class of psychiatric medications.

25. M. Posternak et al., "The Naturalistic Course of Unipolar Major Depression in the Absence of Somatic Therapy," *Journal of Nervous and Mental Disease* 194, no. 5 (May 2006): 324–49.

26. A. Martin et al., "Age Effects on Antidepressant-Induced Manic Conversion," *Archives of Pediatrics and Adolescent Medicine* 158 (August 2002): 773–80.

27. P. S. Jensen et al., "A 3-Year Follow-Up of the NIMH MTA study," *Journal of the American Academy of Child & Adolescent Psychiatry* 46 (August 2007): 989–1002.

28. M. Harrow and T. H. Jobe, "Factors Involved in Outcome and Recovery in Schizophrenia Patients Not on Antipsychotic Medication: A 15-Year Multifollow-Up Study," *Journal of Nervous and Mental Disease* 195, no. 5 (May 2007): 406–14.

29. L. Wunderink et al., "Recovery in Remitted First-Episode Psychosis at 7 Years of Follow-Up of an Early Dose Reduction/Discontinuation or Maintenance Treatment Strategy: Long-Term Follow-Up of a 2-Year Randomized Clinical Trial," *JAMA Psychiatry* 70, no. 9 (September 2013): 913–920. doi:10.1001/jamapsychiatry.2013.19.

30. J. Read and J. Williams, "Adverse Effects of Antidepressants Reported by a Large International Cohort: Emotional Blunting, Suicidality, and Withdrawal Effects," *Current Drug Safety* 13, no. 3 (2018): 176–86. doi: 10.2174/1574886313666180605095130.

31. Y. Lucire and C. Crotty, "Antidepressant-Induced Akathisia-Related Homicides Associated with Diminishing Mutations in Metabolizing Genes of the CYP450 Family," *Pharmacogenomics and Personalized Medicine* 4 (2011): 65–81. doi: 10.2147/PGPM.S17445.

32. Ibid.

33. Sally C. Curtin et al., "Increase in Suicide in the United States, 1999–2014." NCHS Data Brief No. 241, April 2016. https://www.cdc.gov/nchs/products/databriefs/db241.htm.

34. Kim Witczak, "Truth Is . . . We All Could Be Woody," Kelly Brogan M.D. (blog). https://kellybroganmd.com/truth-is-we-all-could-be-woody/.

35. Tanya S. Hauck et al., "ADHD Treatment in Primary Care: Demographic Factors, Medication Trends, and Treatment Predictors," *Canadian Journal of Psychiatry* 62, no. 6 (June 2017): 393–402. doi: 10.1177/0706743716689055.

36. P. Burgess et al., "Do Nations' Mental Health Policies, Programs and Legislation Influence Their Suicide Rates? An Ecological Study of 100 Countries," *Australian and New Zealand Journal of Psychiatry* 38, no. 11–12 (November–December 2004): 933–39.

37. Ajit Ritesh Bhandarkar Shah and Gurleen Bhatia, "The Relationship Between General Population Suicide Rates and Mental Health Funding, Service Provision and National Policy: A Cross-National Study," *International Journal of Social Psychiatry* 56 (August 3, 2009): 448–53. https://doi.org/10.1177/0020764009342384.

38. A. P. Rajkumar et al., "National Suicide Rates and Mental Health System Indicators: An Ecological Study of 191 Countries," *International Journal of Law and Psychiatry*, vol. 36, Issues 5–6 (September–December 2013), 339–42. doi: 10.1016/j.ijlp.2013.06.004.

39. "On Pharma, Corruption, and Psychiatric Drugs," Peter Gøtzsche interview, 11/22/2013, Mad In America website: https://www.madinamerica.com/2013/11/peter-gotzsche-2/.

40. G. A. Fava et al., "Withdrawal Symptoms after Selective Serotonin Reuptake Inhibitor Discontinuation: A Systematic Review," *Psychotherapy and Psychosomatics* 84 (March 2015): 72–81. doi: 10.1159/000370338.

41. Harvard Women's Health Watch, "How to Taper Off Your Antidepressant: Response to Dosage Dictates Best Schedule to Stop Taking Medication," Harvard Health Publishing, Harvard University Medical School, November 2010, updated April 2, 2018, https://www.health.harvard.edu/diseases-and-conditions/how-to-taper-off-your-antidepressant.

42. J. Davies et al., "A Systematic Review into the Incidence, Severity and Duration of Antidepressant Withdrawal Effects: Are Guidelines Evidence-based?" *Addictive Behaviors*, September 18, 2018, https://doi.org/10.1016/j.addbeh.2018.08.027.

43. J. Read et al., "How Many of 1829 Antidepressant Users Report Withdrawal Effects or Addiction?" *International Journal of Mental Health Nursing* 6, no. 27 (June 5, 2018): 1805-15. doi: 10.1111/inm.12488.

44. M. Olfson et al., "Benzodiazepine Use in the United States," *JAMA Psychiatry* 72, no. 2 (February 2015): 136–42. doi: 10.1001/jamapsychiatry.2014.1763.

45. See my blog for details about ingredients, such as gelatin/collagen hydrosylate, coconut oil, and ghee: https://kellybroganmd.com/heres-whats-breakfast-kb -smoothie/.

## Chapter 3: The Point of Pain

1. Francis Weller, *The Wild Edge of Sorrow: Rituals of Renewal and the Sacred Work of Grief* (Berkeley, CA: North Atlantic Books, 2015).

2. Bessel van der Kolk, *The Body Keeps the Score: Brain, Mind, and Body in the Healing of Trauma* (New York: Viking, 2014).

3. See a yogic perspective on releasing childself trauma with useful guided meditation: "Release Childhood Trauma with 3 Min Kundalini Meditation," October 25, 2012. https://www.youtube.com/watch?v=ICfkSHWGqTs.

4. Stephen W. Porges, "The Polyvagal Theory: New Insights into Adaptive Reactions of the Autonomic Nervous System," *Cleveland Clinic Journal of Medicine* 76, Supplement 2 (April 2009): S86–S90. doi: 10.3949/ccjm.76.s2.17.

5. Joseph Aldo's website: http://www.josephaldo.com.

6. Kelly Brogan, "Resolution of Refractory Bipolar Disorder with Psychotic Features and Suicidality Through Lifestyle Interventions: A Case Report," *Advances in Mind-Body Medicine* 31, no. 2 (Spring 2017): 4–11. https://www.ncbi.nlm.nih.gov /pubmed/28659508.

## Chapter 4: Fear Is the Sickness

1. B. R. Rutherford et al., "The Role of Patient Expectancy in Placebo and Nocebo Effects in Antidepressant Trials," *Journal of Clinical Psychiatry* 75, no. 10 (October 2014): 1040–6. doi: 10.4088/JCP.13m08797.

2. Fang Fang et al., "Suicide and Cardiovascular Death after a Cancer Diagnosis," *New England Journal of Medicine* 366 (April 5, 2012) 366: 1310–18. doi: 10.1056 /NEJMoa1110307.

3. Rebecca G. Reed et al., "Emotional Acceptance, Inflammation, and Sickness Symptoms across the First Two Years Following Breast Cancer Diagnosis," *Brain, Behavior, and Immunity* Vol. 56 (August 2016): 165–74. doi: 10.1016/j.bbi.2016 .02.018.

4. A. H. Miller et al., "Neuroendocrine-Immune Mechanisms of Behavioral Comorbidities in Patients with Cancer," *Journal of Clinical Oncology* 20, no. 26 (February 2008): 971–82. doi: 10.1200/JCO.2007.10.7805.

5. M. C. Janelsins et al., "Differential Expression of Cytokines in Breast Cancer Patients Receiving Different Chemotherapies: Implications for Cognitive Impairment Research," *Support Care in Cancer* 20, no. 4 (April 2012): 831–39. doi: 10.1007/s00520-011-1158-0.

6. See her book *Dodging Energy Vampires: An Empath's Guide to Evading Relationships That Drain You and Restoring Your Health and Power* (Hay House, 2018).

7. Gabor Maté, *When the Body Says No: Understanding the Stress-Disease Connection* (Hoboken, NJ: John Wiley & Sons, 2003).

8. John R. Strachan, *A Routledge Literary Sourcebook on the Poems of John Keats* (New York: Routledge, 2003).

9. Lisa Bloomquist, "What is Fluoroquinolone Toxicity?," *Hormones Matter*, May 25, 2015. https://www.hormonesmatter.com/fluoroquinolone-toxicity/.

10. W. J. Sng and D. Y. Wang, "Efficacy and Side Effects of Antibiotics in the Treatment of Acute Rhinosinusitis: A Systematic Review," *Rhinology* 53, no. 1 (March 2015): 3–9. doi: 10.4193/Rhin13.225.

11. L. C. McDonald et al., "Effects of Short- and Long-Course Antibiotics on the Lower Intestinal Microbiome as They Relate to Traveller's Diarrhea," *Journal of Travel Medicine* 1, no. 24 (supplement 1) (April 2017): S35-S38. doi: 10.1093/jtm/taw084.

12. L. Dethlefsen et al., "The Pervasive Effects of an Antibiotic on the Human Gut Microbiota, as Revealed by Deep 16S rRNA Sequencing," *PLoS Biology* 18, no. 6 (11) (November 2008): e280. doi: 10.1371/journal.pbio.0060280.

13. F. Guarner and J. R. Malagelada, "Gut Flora in Health and Disease," *Lancet* 8, no. 361 (9356) (February 2003): 512–19. doi: 10.1016/S0140-6736(03)12489-0.

14. H. Tlaskalová-Hogenová et al., "Commensal Bacteria (Normal Microflora), Mucosal Immunity and Chronic Inflammatory and Autoimmune Diseases," *Immunology Letters* 15, no. 93 (2–3) (May 2004): 97–108. doi: 10.1016/j.imlet.2004.02.005.

15. Peter J. Turnbaugh et al., "An Obesity-associated Gut Microbiome with Increased Capacity for Energy Harvest," *Nature* 444 (December 21, 2006), 1027–31.

16. I. Tuncay et al., "A Comparison of Effects of Fluoroquinolones on Fracture Healing (an Experimental Study in Rats)," Ulusal travma ve acil cerrahi dergisi/ *Turkish Journal of Trauma and Emergency Surgery* 11, no. 1 (January 2005): 17–22. PMID: 15688263.

17. J. M. Paterson et al., "Fluoroquinolone Therapy and Idiosyncratic Acute Liver Injury: A Population-Based Study," *Canadian Medical Association Journal* 2, no. 184 (14) (October 2012): 1565–70. doi: 10.1503/cmaj.111823.

18. Stig Bengmark, "Gut Microbiota, Immune Development and Function," *Pharmacological Research* 69, Issue 1 (March 2013) 87–113. doi: 10.1016/j.phrs.2012.09.002.

19. German New Medicine is not only a new paradigm of medicine, but also a new consciousness. It is the awareness that our organism possesses inexhaustible creativity and remarkable self-healing capabilities. It is the recognition that each cell of our body is endowed with biological wisdom we share with all living beings. See his website for more info: https://learninggnm.com.

20. Fang Fang, "Suicide and Cardiovascular Death after a Cancer Diagnosis."

21. W. Lorber, G. Manzzoni, and I. Kirsch, "Illness by Suggestion: Expectancy, Modeling, and Gender in the Production of Psychosomatic Symptoms," *Annals of Behavioral Medicine* 33, no. 1 (February 2007): 112–16. doi: 10.1207/s15324796abm3301_13.

22. Charles Eisenstein, *The Ascent of Humanity: Civilization and the Human Sense of Self* (Berkeley, CA: Evolver Editions, 2013).

23.  Happy, Healthy, Holy Organization, "Meditation for a Calm Heart." https://
     www.3ho.org/kundalini-yoga/pranayam/pranayam-techniques/meditation
     -calm-heart.

## Chapter 5: From Mess to Meaning: Five Psychiatric "Pretenders"

1.   Huai Heng Loh et al., "Association between Subclinical Hypothyroidism and
     Depression: An Updated Systematic Review and Meta-Analysis," *BMC Psychiatry*
     19 (January 8, 2019): 12. doi: 10.1186/s12888-018-2006-2.

2.   D. Bernardo et al., "Is Gliadin Really Safe for Non-Coeliac Individuals?" *Gut* 56,
     no. 6 (June 2007): 889–90. doi: 10.1136/gut.2006.118265

3.   H. K. Delichatsios et al., "Case 14-2016—A 37-Year-Old Woman with Adult-Onset
     Psychosis," *New England Journal of Medicine* 374 (May 12, 2016): 1875–83. doi:
     10.1056/NEJMcpc1514473.

4.   A. Fasano, "Leaky Gut and Autoimmune Diseases," *Clinical Reviews in Allergy and
     Immunology* 42, no. 1 (February 2012): 71–8. doi: 10.1007/s12016-011-8291-x.

5.   Sayer Ji, "60 Years of Research Links Gluten Grains to Schizophrenia,"
     GreenMedInfo, August 27, 2018. http://www.greenmedinfo.com/blog/60-years
     -research-links-gluten-grains-schizophrenia.

6.   O. Olaoluwa et al., "Elevated Gliadin Antibody Levels in Individuals with
     Schizophrenia," *World Journal of Biological Psychiatry* 14, no. 7 (September 2013):
     509–15. doi: 10.3109/15622975.2012.747699.

7.   E. G. Severance et al., "Subunit and Whole Molecule Specificity of the Anti-
     Bovine Casein Immune Response in Recent Onset Psychosis and Schizophrenia,"
     *Schizophrenia Research* 118, no. 1–3 (May 2010): 240–47. doi: 10.1016/j.schres
     .2009.12.030. Epub 2010 Jan 13.

8.   Suzanne M. de la Monte and Jack R. Wands, "Alzheimer's Disease Is Type 3
     Diabetes—Evidence Reviewed," *Journal of Diabetes Science and Technology* 2, no. 6
     (November 2008): 1101–13. doi: 10.1177/193229680800200619.

9.   M. A. Fishel et al., "Hyperinsulinemia Provokes Synchronous Increases in Central
     Inflammation and Beta-Amyloid in Normal Adults," *Archives of Neurology* 62, no.
     10 (October 2005): 1539–44. doi: 10.1001/archneur.62.10.noc50112.

10.  N. Berry et al., "Catatonia and Other Psychiatric Symptoms with Vitamin B12
     Deficiency," *Acta Psychiatrica Scandinavica* 108, no. 2 (August 2003): 156–59.
     PMID: 12823174.

11.  Judy McBride, "B12 Deficiency May Be More Widespread Than Thought," USDA
     Agricultural Research Service, August 2, 2000. https://www.ars.usda.gov/news-
     events/news/research-news/2000/b12-deficiency-may-be-more-widespread-than
     -thought/.

12.  J. R. Lam et al., "Proton Pump Inhibitor and Histamine 2 Receptor Antagonist
     Use and Vitamin B12 Deficiency," *Journal of the American Medical Association* 310,
     no. 22 (December 11, 2013): 2435–42. doi:10.1001/jama.2013.280490.

13.  Mayo News Releases, "Nearly 7 in 10 Americans Take Prescription Drugs, Mayo
     Clinic, Olmsted Medical Center Find," Mayo News Network, June 19, 2013,
     https://newsnetwork.mayoclinic.org/discussion/nearly-7-in-10-americans-take
     -prescription-drugs-mayo-clinic-olmsted-medical-center-find/.

14.  Teresa Carr, "Too Many Meds? America's Love Affair with Prescription
     Medication," *Consumer Reports*, October 3, 2017, https://www.consumerreports.
     org/prescription-drugs/too-many-meds-americas-love-affair-with-prescription
     -medication/.

15.  D. M. Qato et al., "Prevalence of Prescription Medications with Depression as a Potential Adverse Effect Among Adults in the United States," *Journal of the American Medical Association* 319, no. 22 (June 12, 2018): 2289. doi: 10.1001/jama.2018.6741.

16.  J. Kulkarni, "Depression as a Side Effect of the Contraceptive Pill," *Expert Opinion on Drug Safety* 6, no. 4 (July 2007): 371–74. doi: 10.1517/14740338.6.4.371.

17.  K. A. Oinonen et al., "To What Extent Do Oral Contraceptives Influence Mood and Affect?" *Journal of Affective Disorders* 70, no. 3 (August 2002): 229–40. PMID: 12128235.

18.  C. W. Skovlund et al., "Association of Hormonal Contraception with Depression," *JAMA Psychiatry* 73 (November 1, 2016): 1154–62. doi: 10.1001/jamapsychiatry .2016.2387.

19.  C. W. Skovlund et al., "Association of Hormonal Contraception with Suicide Attempts and Suicides," *Psychiatry* 175, no. 4 (April 2018): 336–42. doi: 10.1176 /appi.ajp.2017.17060616.

20.  M. Sokolowski, J. Wasserman, and D. Wasserman, "An overview of the Neurobiology of Suicidal Behaviors as One Meta-System," *Molecular Psychiatry* 20, no. 1 (February 2015): 56–71. doi: 10.1038/mp.2014.101.

21.  John Michael Bostwick and V. Shane Pankratz, "Affective Disorders and Suicide Risk: A Reexamination," *American Journal of Psychiatry* 157, no. 12 (December 1, 2000): 1925–32. https://doi.org/10.1176/appi.ajp.157.12.1925.

22.  H. Zhang et al, "Discontinuation of Statins in Routine Care Settings: Cohort Study," *Annals of Internal Medicine* 158, no. 7 (April 2, 2013): 526–34. doi: 10.7326/0003-4819-158-7-201304020-00004.

23.  Vesza, Zsófia, Catarina Pires, and Pedro Marques da Silva, "Statin-Related Lichenoid Dermatosis: An Uncommon Adverse Reaction to a Common Treatment," *European Journal of Case Reports in Internal Medicine* 5, no. 5 (May 2018): 000844. doi: 10.12890/2018_000844.

24.  M. Virkkunen, "Serum cholesterol levels in homicidal offenders. A low cholesterol level is connected with a habitually violent tendency under the influence of alcohol," *Neuropsychobiology* 10, no. 2–3 (1983): 65–69. doi: 10.1159/000117987.

25.  See numerous studies as reported on greenmed.com, http://www.greenmedinfo .com/greenmed/topic/47443/focus/856/page.

26.  M. Tuccori et al., "Neuropsychiatric Adverse Events Associated with Statins: Epidemiology, Pathophysiology, Prevention and Management," *CNS Drugs* 28, no. 3 (March 2014): 249–72. doi: 10.1007/s40263-013-0135-1.

27.  David M. Diamond and Uffe Ravnskov, "How Statistical Deception Created the Appearance That Statins Are Safe and Effective in Primary and Secondary Prevention of Cardiovascular Disease," *Expert Review of Clinical Pharmacology* 8, no. 2 (March 2015): 201. doi: 10.1586/17512433.2015.1012494.

28.  Qato et al., "Prevalence of Prescription Medications with Depression as a Potential Adverse Effect Among Adults in the United States." Some of those 200-plus medications are also available over the counter (OTC).

29.  Carr, "Too Many Meds? America's Love Affair with Prescription Medication."

30.  T. Christian Miller and Jeff Gerth, "Behind the Numbers: We Explore the Data Behind Figures Showing How Many People Die from Overdosing on Acetaminophen, the Active Ingredient in Tylenol," *ProPublica*, September 20, 2013. https://www.propublica.org/article/tylenol-mcneil-fda-behind-the-numbers.

31.  Carmen Drahl, "How Does Acetaminophen Work? Researchers Still Aren't Sure," *Chemical and Engineering News* 92, Issue 29 (July 21, 2014): 31–32. https://cen.acs .org/articles/92/i29/Does-Acetaminophen-Work-Researchers-Still.html.

32. John T. Slattery et al., "Dose-Dependent Pharmacokinetics of Acetaminophen: Evidence of Glutathione Depletion in Humans," *Clinical Pharmacology and Therapeutics* 41, no. 4 (April 1987): 413–18. doi:10.1038/clpt.1987.50.

33. R. O. Geoffrey et al., "Over-the-Counter Relief from Pains and Pleasures Alike: Acetaminophen Blunts Evaluation Sensitivity to Both Negative and Positive Stimuli," *Psychological Science* 26, no. 6 (April 10, 2015): 750–58. doi: 10.1177/0956797615570366.

34. European League Against Rheumatism, "Non-Steroidal Anti-Inflammatory Drugs Inhibit Ovulation after Just 10 Days," *ScienceDaily*, June 11, 2015. www .sciencedaily.com/releases/2015/06/150611082124.htm.

35. D. Y. Graham et al., "Visible Small-Intestinal Mucosal Injury in Chronic NSAID Users," *Clinical Gastroenterology and Hepatology* 3, no. 1 (January 2005): 55–59. PMID: 15645405.

36. G. Sigthorsson et al., "Intestinal Permeability and Inflammation in Patients on NSAIDs," *Gut* 43, no. 4 (October 1998): 506–11. PMID: 9824578.

37. H. Sternbach and R. State, "Antibiotics: Neuropsychiatric Effects and Psychotropic Interactions," *Harvard Review of Psychiatry* 5, no. 4 (November–December 1997): 214–26. https://www.ncbi.nlm.nih.gov/pubmed/9427014.

38. N. Zareifopoulos and G. Panayiotakopoulos, "Neuropsychiatric Effects of Antimicrobial Agents," *Clinical Drug Investigation* 37 (May 2017): 423. https:// www.ncbi.nlm.nih.gov/pubmed/28197902.

39. S. Lambrichts et al., "Antibiotics and Mania: A Systematic Review," *Journal of Affective Disorders* 219 (September 2017): 149–56. doi: 10.1016/j.jad.2017.05.029.

40. Nora Hamdani et al., "Resolution of a Manic Episode Treated with Activated Charcoal: Evidence for a Brain-Gut Axis in Bipolar Disorder," *Australian and New Zealand Journal of Psychiatry* 49, no. 12 (December 2015): 1221–13. doi: 10.1177/0004867415595873.

41. I. Lurie et al., "Antibiotic Exposure and the Risk for Depression, Anxiety, or Psychosis: A Nested Case-Control Study," *Journal of Clinical Psychiatry* 76, no. 11 (November 2015): 1522–28. doi: 10.4088/JCP.15m09961.

42. To access a user-friendly, comprehensive resource center on the effects of vaccines and, in particular, the reporting of adverse reactions, visit the National Vaccine information Center at http://medalerts.org/. I have written extensively on my concerns about vaccines, especially in vulnerable populations. I invite you to visit my website and use its search function to read more about my stand on vaccines and the supporting studies.

43. See my post "A Scientist Speaks: Senate Bill 277 in California" at www. kellybroganmd.com, May 7, 2015, http://kellybroganmd.com/article/scientist -speaks-senate-bill-277-california/.

44. For more information about dangers of vaccines, see my e-book Special Report: *Vaccines and Brain Health*, available from my website.

45. See the website https://usa.daysy.me for how to purchase.

46. V. Kuptniratsaikul et al., "Efficacy and Safety of Curcuma domestica Extracts in Patients with Knee Osteoarthritis," *Journal of Alternative and Complementary Medicine* 15, no. 8 (August 2009): 891–97. doi: 10.1089/acm.2008.0186.

47. G. Ozgoli et al., "Comparison of Effects of Ginger, Mefenamic Acid, and Ibuprofen on Pain in Women with Primary Dysmenorrhea," *Journal of Alternative and Complementary Medicine* 15, no. 2 (February 2009): 129–32. doi: 10.1089/ acm.2008.0311.

## Chapter 6: A Reunion with Your Body in One Month

1. F. N. Jacka et al., "Red Meat Consumption and Mood and Anxiety Disorders," *Psychotherapy and Psychosomatics* 81, no. 3 (March 2012): 196–98. doi: 10.1159/000334910.

2. See the Environmental Working Group (EWG) website for a list of the 2018 Dirty Dozen: EWG's 2018 Shopper's Guide to Pesticides in Produce, https://www.ewg .org/foodnews/dirty-dozen.php#.WeTVfmhSxPZ. White potatoes are on this list but are not a part of the Reset diet.

3. G. Den Besten et al., "The Role of Short-Chain Fatty Acids in the Interplay Between Diet, Gut Microbiota, and Host Energy Metabolism," *Journal of Lipid Research* 54, no. 9 (September 2013): 2325–40. doi: 10.1194/jlr.R036012.

4. J. Slavin et al., "Fiber and Prebiotics: Mechanisms and Health Benefits," *Nutrients* 5, no. 4 (April 22, 2013): 1417–35. doi: 10.3390/nu5041417.

5. K. L. Johnston et al., "Resistant Starch Improves Insulin Sensitivity in Metabolic Syndrome," *Diabetic Medicine* 27, no. 4 (April 2010): 391–97. doi: 10.1111/j.1464 -5491.2010.02923.x.

6. See www.localfarmmarkets.org for more information.

7. J. R. Barrett, "Chemical Exposures: The Ugly Side of Beauty Products," *Environmental Health Perspectives* 113, no. 1 (January 2005): A24. doi: 10.1289/ehp.113-a24.

8. U.S. Food and Drug Administration, "FDA Authority Over Cosmetics: How Cosmetics Are Not FDA-Approved, but Are FDA-Regulated." March 3, 2005, last updated July 24, 2018. https://www.fda.gov/cosmetics/guidanceregulation /lawsregulations/ucm074162.htm.

9. Barrett, "Chemical Exposures: The Ugly Side of Beauty Products."

10. Two websites for checking products' safety ratings can be found: EWG's Skin Deep, https://www.ewg.org/skindeep/, and I Read Labels for You, https:// ireadlabelsforyou.com/.

11. Go to Wellness Mama, 7 Ingredients—20+ DIY Natural Beauty Recipes, https:// wellnessmama.com/5801/diy-beauty-recipes/.

12. C. Stajano, "The Concentrated Coffee Enema in the Therapeutics of Shock," *Uruguayan Medical, Surgical and Specialization Archives* 29 (1941): 1–27.

13. "Bedside procedures" in *The Merck Manual of Diagnosis and Therapy, 11th ed.,* ed. C. E. Lyght et al. (Rahway, NJ: Merck Sharp & Dohme Research Laboratories, 1966), 1682–83.

14. A. L. Garbat and H. G. Jacobi, "Secretion of Bile in Response to Rectal Installations," *Archives of Internal Medicine* 44 (1929): 455–62.

15. A. Goshvarpour and A. Goshvarpour, "Comparison of Higher Order Spectra in Heart Rate Signals During Two Techniques of Meditation: Chi and Kundalini Meditation," *Cognitive Neurodynamics* 7, no. 1 (February 2012): 39–46. doi: 10.1007/s11571-012-9215-z.

16. M. Engström et al., "Functional Magnetic Resonance Imaging of Hippocampal Activation During Silent Mantra Meditation," *Journal of Alternative and Complementary Medicine* 16, no. 12 (December 2010): 1253–58. doi: 10.1089 /acm.2009.0706.

17. D. S. Shannahoff-Khalsa et al., "Randomized Controlled Trial of Yogic Meditation Techniques for Patients with Obsessive-Compulsive Disorder," *CNS Spectrums* 4, no. 12 (December 1999): 34–47. PMID: 18311106.

18. D. S. Shannahoff-Khalsa, "An Introduction to Kundalini Yoga Meditation

Techniques That Are Specific for the Treatment of Psychiatric Disorders," *Journal of Alternative and Complementary Medicine* 10, no. 1 (February 2004): 91–101. doi: 10.1089/107555304322849011.

19. See Alzheimer's Research and Prevention Foundation, http://alzheimersprevention.org/research/journal-articles/.

20. See my website, https://kellybroganmd.com/downloads/, for a free, video-based download of starter meditations to commit to for 3 minutes a day.

21. For more info and a discount code for classes, go to http://KukuwaFitness.com/WorkOutOnline KBMD10.

22. E. Lee et al., "Persistent Sleep Disturbance: A Risk Factor for Recurrent Depression in Community-Dwelling Older Adults," *Sleep* 36, no. 11 (November 1, 2013): 1685–91. doi:10.5665/sleep.3128.

23. C. L. Raison et al., "Chronic Interferon-Alpha Administration Disrupts Sleep Continuity and Depth in Patients with Hepatitis C: Association with Fatigue, Motor Slowing, and Increased Evening Cortisol," *Biological Psychiatry* 68, no. 10 (November 15, 2010): 942–49. doi: 10.1016/j.biopsych.2010.04.019.

24. H. Woelk and S. Schläfke, "A Multi-Center, Double-Blind, Randomised Study of the Lavender Oil Preparation Silexan in Comparison to Lorazepam for Generalized Anxiety Disorder," *Phytomedicine* 17, Issue 2 (February 2010): 94–99. doi: 10.1016/j.phymed.2009.10.006.

## Chapter 7: Moving beyond Meds and Navigating the Dark Night

1. His website is https://breggin.com.

2. G. A. Fava et al., "Withdrawal Symptoms after Selective Serotonin Reuptake Inhibitor Discontinuation: A Systematic Review," *Psychotherapy and Psychosomatics* 84 (March 2015): 72–81. doi: 10.1159/000370338.

3. G. Chouinard and V. A. Chouinard, "New Classification of Selective Serotonin Reuptake Inhibitor Withdrawal," *Psychotherapy and Psychosomatics* 84 (2015): 63–71. doi: 10.1159/000371865.

4. Jonathan E. Prousky, "Tapering Off Psychotropic Drugs: Using Patient Cases to Understand Reasons for Success and Failure," *Journal of Orthomolecular Medicine* 28, no. 4 (2013): 159–74. http://psychrights.org/research/digest/Wthdrawal/Tapering_Success_and_FailureJProusky2013.pdf.

5. James Davies and John Read, "A Systematic Review into the Incidence, Severity and Duration of Antidepressant Withdrawal Effects: Are Guidelines Evidence-Based?," *Addictive Behavior* (September 4, 2018) pii: S0306-4603(18)30834-7. doi: 10.1016/j.addbeh.2018.08.027.

6. T. Stockmann et al., "SSRI and SNRI Withdrawal Symptoms Reported on an Internet Forum," *International Journal of Risk and Safety in Medicine* 29, no. 3–4 (2018): 175–80. doi: 10.3233/JRS-180018.

7. See Heartmath.com.

8. For more detail, go to traumacenter.org.

9. If you don't have a supportive clinician (and even if you do), https://www.theinnercompass.org/ is a powerful and informative resource.

10. Robert Whitaker, Robert, "Making the Case Against Antidepressants in Parliament," Mad in America (May 10, 2016). https://www.madinamerica.com/2016/05/making-the-case-against-antidepressants-in-parliament/.

11. See IONS.org for distance healing studies and articles.

12. A. Winokur et al., "The Effects of Antidepressants on Sleep," *Psychiatric Times* 29, no. 6 (June 13, 2012). https://www.psychiatrictimes.com/effects-antidepressants -sleep/.

13. Yetish, G., et al., "Natural Sleep and Its Seasonal Variations in Three Pre-industrial Societies," *Current Biology* 25, Issue 21 (November 2, 2015): P2862–68. doi: 10.1016/j.cub.2015.09.046.

14. Resource: See Lotuswei.com for my dear friend Katie Hess's own line of flower essences, Lotus Wei (lotuswei.com), in the form of elixirs, mists, skin serums, and natural perfumes that are focused on joy, pleasure, expansion, and invoking exalted feelings; they are a staple in my energetic toolkit.

15. Resource: For a free app to get you started, go to https://www .thetappingsolutionapp.com/.

## Chapter 8: The Lens of Your Perception

1. A. Ray et al., "Stress, Anxiety, and Immunomodulation: A Pharmacological Analysis," *Vitamins and Hormones* 103 (2017): 1–25. doi: 10.1016 /bs.vh.2016.09.007.

2. B. S. McEwen, "Stress, Adaptation, and Disease. Allostasis and Allostatic Load," *Annals of the New York Academy of Sciences* 840 (May 1, 1998): 33–44. PMID: 9629234.

3. S. Cohen et al., "Self-Rated Health in Healthy Adults and Susceptibility to the Common Cold," *Psychosomatic Medicine* 77, no. 9 (November–December 2015): 959–68. doi: 10.1097/PSY.0000000000000232.

4. Vanda Faria et al., "Do You Believe It? Verbal Suggestions Influence the Clinical and Neural Effects of Escitalopram in Social Anxiety Disorder: A Randomized Trial," *EBioMedicine* 24 (October 2017): 179–88. doi: 10.1016/j.ebiom.2017.09.031.

5. A. Hampshire et al., "The Role of the Right Inferior Frontal Gyrus: Inhibition and Attentional Control," *Neuroimage* 50, no. 3 (April 15, 2010): 1313–19. doi: 10.1016/j.neuroimage.2009.12.109.

6. T. L. Ferreira et al., "The Indirect Amygdala–Dorsal Striatum Pathway Mediates Conditioned Freezing: Insights on Emotional Memory Networks," *Neuroscience* 153, Issue 1 (April 22, 2008): 84–94. doi: 10.1016/j.neuroscience.2008.02.013.

7. C. S. Ginandes et al., "Using Hypnosis to Accelerate the Healing of Bone Fractures: A Randomized Controlled Pilot Study," *Alternative Therapies in Health and Medicine* 5, no. 2 (March 1999): 67–75.

8. See Dr. Sheldrake's website, Sheldrake.org (https://www.sheldrake.org/research /morphic-resonance).

9. Rupert Sheldrake, *The Science Delusion* (London: Hodder & Stoughton, 2012).

10. See Dr. Bland's 30-minute keynote entitled "Genetic Dark Matter: Decoding the Force Within" at https://functionalforum.com/march-2016-functional-forum.

11. King, M. et al., "Breast and Ovarian Cancer Risks Due to Inherited Mutations in BRCA1 and BRCA," *Science* 302 (5645) (October 24, 2003): 643–46.

12. Alexandra J. van den Broek et al., "Worse Breast Cancer Prognosis of BRCA1/ BRCA2 Mutation Carriers: What's the Evidence? A Systematic Review with Meta-Analysis," *PLOS One* 10, no. 3 (March 27, 2015): e0120189. doi: 10.1371/journal .pone.0120189.

13. From "Swimming Headless" in Watts, Alan, *Eastern Wisdom, Modern Life: Collected Talks 1960–1969* (Novato, CA: New World Library, 2006).

14. Healthy, Happy, Holy Organization, "Two-Stroke Breath to Connect the Subconscious and the Intuition." https://www.3ho.org/kundalini-yoga/pranayam /two-stroke-breath-connect-subconscious-and-intuition.

## Chapter 9: Coming Home to You

1. See website: https://www.heartmath.org/research/.

2. Visit Louise Hay's foundation website, https://www.louisehay.com, for more about her.

3. For more information, visit https://homesweethomebirth.com/clarity-breathwork -new-york.

4. For the Cutting Cords Meditation recording, go to https://kellybroganmd.com /cutting-cords-meditation/.

5. See his essay, adapted from a talk he gave to the California Institute of Integral Studies in 2008, at ScienceAndDuality.com: https://www.scienceandnonduality .com/intimate-relationship-as-a-spiritual-crucible.

6. S. R. H. Beach et al., "When Inflammation and Depression Go Together: The Longitudinal Effects of Parent-Child Relationships," *Developmental Psychopathology* 29, no. 5 (December 2017): 1969–86. doi: 10.1017 /S0954579417001523.

7. Ajay Abraham et al., "The Effect of Mobile Phone Use on Prosocial Behavior," *ResearchGate*, 2019. https://www.researchgate.net/publication/267687748_The _Effect_of_Mobile_Phone_Use_on_Prosocial_Behavior.

8. Bruce K. Alexander, "Addiction: The View from Rat Park (2010)," 2010. For articles on his studies, see his website, http://www.brucekalexander.com.

9. S. W. Cole et al., "Loneliness, Eudaimonia, and the Human Conserved Transcriptional Response to Adversity," *Psychoneuroendocrinology* 62 (December 2015): 11–17. doi: 10.1016/j.psyneuen.2015.07.001.

10. See website: https://www.chicenter.com.

11. Mington Gu, "How to Heal with Light Ball—Wisdom Healing Qigong" (February 12, 2014). https://www.youtube.com/watch?v=m4JcTVd9Tv4.

12. Neale Donald Walsch, *Conversations with God* (New York: G. P. Putnam's Sons, 1996).

## Chapter 10: Faith: Trust in a Grand Design

1. Her website is http://www.joanborysenko.com, and you can see more of her books and classes at www.hayhouse.com.

2. See Emma Bragdon's website, https://imhu.org/, and https://www.emmabragdon .com/ for more about her writing and her two documentary films on the relationship between spirituality and health. She also teaches the online course "How to Effectively Support Someone in Spiritual Emergency," trains and certifies Spiritual Emergence Coaches, and leads a weeklong seminar in Brazil once a year for health care providers wanting to learn more about Spiritist therapies. IMHU is currently raising money to produce films to educate health care providers and the general public about spiritual emergency.

3. Malidoma Somé can be reached through his website, http://malidoma.com /main/. He teaches widely and continues to offer personal consultations. He is also the author of several books that illuminate his wisdom about shamanic initiation, ritual, and community.

4. A. S. Junior et al., "William James and Psychical Research: Towards a Radical Science of Mind," *History of Psychiatry* 24, no. 1 (March 2013): 62–78. doi:10.1177/0957154X12450138.

5. B. Q. Ford et al., "The Psychological Health Benefits of Accepting Negative Emotions and Thoughts: Laboratory, Diary, and Longitudinal Evidence," *Journal of Personality and Social Psychology* 115, no. 6 (December 2018): 1075–92. doi: 10.1037/pspp0000157.

6. See my e-book *Psychedelics and Mental Health*, available as a free PDF download on my website.

7. Michael Pollan, *How to Change Your Mind: What the New Science of Psychedelics Teaches Us About Consciousness, Dying, Addiction, Depression, and Transcendence* (New York: Penguin, 2019).

8. E. Domínguez-Clavé et al., "Ayahuasca: Pharmacology, Neuroscience and Therapeutic Potential," *Brain Research Bulletin* 126, pt. 1 (September 2016): 89–101. doi: 10.1016/j.brainresbull.2016.03.002.

9. R. G. Dos Santos et al., "Antidepressive and Anxiolytic Effects of Ayahuasca: A Systematic Literature Review of Animal and Human Studies," *Brazilian Journal of Psychiatry* (Revista Brasileira de Psiciatria) 38, no. 1 (March 2016): 65–72. doi: 10.1590/1516-4446-2015-1701.

10. J. J. Rucker et al., "Psychedelics in the Treatment of Unipolar Mood Disorders: A Systematic Review," *Journal of Psychopharmacology* (Oxford, U.K.) 30, no. 12 (December 2016): 1220–29. Epub 2016 Nov 17.

11. Charles L. Raison, "Everything Old Is New Again: Are Psychedelic Medicines Poised to Take Mental Health by Storm?" *Acta Psychiatrica Scandinavica* 138 (November 2018): 365–67. doi: 10.1111/acps.12975.

12. J. Soler et al., "Exploring the Therapeutic Potential of Ayahuasca: Acute Intake Increases Mindfulness-Related Capacities," *Psychopharmacology* (Berlin) 233, no. 5 (March 2016): 823–29. doi: 10.1007/s00213-015-4162-0.

13. K. P. Kuypers et al., "Ayahuasca Enhances Creative Divergent Thinking While Decreasing Conventional Convergent Thinking," *Psychopharmacology* (Berlin) 233, no. 18 (September 2016): 3395–403. doi: 10.1007/s00213-016-4377-8.

14. M. Forstmann and C. Sagioglou, "Lifetime Experience with (Classic) Psychedelics Predicts Pro-Environmental Behavior Through an Increase in Nature Relatedness," *Journal of Psychopharmacology* (Oxford, U.K.) 31, no. 8 (August 2017): 975–88. doi: 10.1177/0269881117714049.

15. B. J. Park et al., "The Physiological Effects of Shinrin-yoku (Taking in the Forest Atmosphere or Forest Bathing): Evidence from Field Experiments in 24 Forests across Japan," *Environmental Health and Preventive Medicine* 15, no. 1 (January 2010): 18–26. doi: 10.1007/s12199-009-0086-9.

16. G. Chevalier et al., "Earthing: Health Implications of Reconnecting the Human Body to the Earth's Surface Electrons," *Journal of Environmental and Public Health* 2012 (January 12, 2012): 291541. PMID: 22291721.

17. For more information, go to: https://www.dhamma.org/en-US/index.

18. White Tantric Yoga: The Workshop, https://www.whitetantricyoga.com/pages /workshop.

19. For research data see: http://chicenter.com-research-data-for-health-care-pros
    .pages.ontraport.net.

20. Resource for contact information: https://www.chicenter.com/Chi/Home/index
    .cfm?&app=chicenter&ssl=set.

21. For more information: Grof Transpersonal Training, "About Holotropic Breathwork."
    http://www.holotropic.com/holotropic-breathwork/about-holotropic-breathwork/.

## Appendix A

1. Alfie Kohn, *Unconditional Parenting: Moving from Rewards and Punishments to Love
   and Reason* (New York: Atria, 2005).

2. Ibid.

3. Ibid.

4. Ibid.

5. For more information on Natalie and her work, visit her website: https://www
   .centerforemotionaleducation.com.

## Appendix B

1. J. J. Guo et al., "The anti-Staphylococcus aureus Activity of the Phenanthrene
   Fraction from Fibrous Roots of Bletilla striata," *BMC Complementary and Alternative
   Medicine* 1 (November 29, 2016): 491. doi: 10.1186/s12906-016-1488-z.

2. V. Chedid et al., "Herbal Therapy Is Equivalent to Rifaximin for the Treatment of
   Small Intestinal Bacterial Overgrowth," *Global Advances in Health and Medicine* 3,
   no. 3 (May 2014): 16–24. doi: 10.7453/gahmj.2014.019.

3. B. Fu et al., "Inhibition of Pseudomonas aeruginosa Biofilm Formation
   by Traditional Chinese Medicinal Herb Herba patriniae," *Biomed Research
   International* 2017, no. 136 (March 9, 2017): Article 9584703. doi:
   10.1155/2017/9584703.

4. S. O'Shea et al, "In Vitro Activity of Inula helenium Against Clinical
   Staphylococcus aureus Strains Including MRSA," *British Journal of Biomedical
   Science* 66, no. 4 (2009): 186–89. PMID: 20095126.

5. C. Latha et al., "Antiplasmid Activity of 1'-Acetoxychavicol Acetate from Alpinia
   galanga Against Multi-Drug Resistant Bacteria," *Journal of Ethnopharmacology* 123,
   no. 3 (June 25, 2009): 522–25. doi: 10.1016/j.jep.2009.03.028.

6. A. Hannan and S. Saleem, "Anti Bacterial Activity of Nigella sativa Against
   Clinical Isolates of Methicillin Resistant Staphylococcus aureus," *Journal of
   Ayub Medical College, Abbottabad* 20, no. 3 (July–September 2008): 72–74. PMID:
   19610522.

7. S. Ravishankar et al., "Plant-Derived Compounds Inactivate Antibiotic-Resistant
   Campylobacter jejuni Strains," *Journal of Food Protection* 71, no. 6 (June 2008):
   1145–49.

8. S. Derakhshan et al., "Effect of Cumin (Cuminum cyminum) Seed Essential
   Oil on Biofilm Formation and Plasmid Integrity of Klebsiella pneumoniae,"
   *Pharmacognosy Magazine* 6, no. 21 (January 2010): 57–61. doi: 10.4103/0973
   -1296.59967.

9. S. Luqman et al., "Potential of Rosemary Oil to Be Used in Drug-Resistant
   Infections," *Alternative Therapies in Health and Medicine* 13, no. 5 (September–
   October 2007): 54–59. PMID: 17900043.

10. R. S. Porter and R. F. Bode, "A Review of the Antiviral Properties of Black Elder (Sambucus nigra L.) Products," *Phytotherapy Research* 31, no. 4 (April 2017): 533–54. doi: 10.1002/ptr.5782.

11. A. Salehzadeh et al., "Antimicrobial Activity of Methanolic Extracts of Sambucus ebulus and Urtica dioica Against Clinical Isolates of Methicillin Resistant Staphylococcus aureus," *African Journal of Traditional Complementary and Alternative Medicine* 11, no. 5 (August 23, 2014): 38–40. PMID: 25395702.

12. H. Sakkas and C. Papadopoulou, "Antimicrobial Activity of Basil, Oregano, and Thyme Essential Oils," *Journal of Microbiology and Biotechnology* 27, no. 3 (March 28, 2017):429–38. doi: 10.4014/jmb.1608.08024.

13. J. Coccimiglio. et al., "Antioxidant, Antibacterial, and Cytotoxic Activities of the Ethanolic Origanum vulgare Extract and Its Major Constituents," *Oxidative Medicine and Cellular Longevity* 2 (2016): 1–8. doi: 10.1155/2016/1404505.

14. A. Schapowal et al., "Echinacea/Sage or Chlorhexidine/Lidocaine for Treating Acute Sore Throats: A Randomized Double-Blind Trial," *European Journal of Medical Research* 14, no. 9 (September 1, 2009): 406–12. PMID: 19748859.

15. W. Weber et al., "Echinacea purpurea for Prevention of Upper Respiratory Tract Infections in Children," *Journal of Alternative and Complementary Medicine* 11, no. 6 (December 2005): 1021–26. doi: 10.1089/acm.2005.11.1021.

16. D. M. et al., "In Vitro Effects of Echinacea and Ginseng on Natural Killer and Antibody-Dependent Cell Cytotoxicity in Healthy Subjects and Chronic Fatigue Syndrome or Acquired Immunodeficiency Syndrome Patients," *Immunopharmacology* 35, no. 3 (January 1997): 229–35. PMID: 9043936.

17. N. B. Cech et al., "Quorum Quenching and Antimicrobial Activity of Goldenseal (Hydrastis canadensis) Against Methicillin-Resistant Staphylococcus aureus (MRSA)," *Planta Medica* 78, no. 4 (September 2012): 1556–61. doi: 10.1055/s-0032-1315042.

18. G. B. Mahady et al., "In Vitro Susceptibility of Helicobacter pylori to Isoquinoline Alkaloids from Sanguinaria canadensis and Hydrastis canadensis," *Phytotherapy Research* 17, no. 3 (March 2003): 217–21. doi: 10.1002/ptr.1108.

19. F. Scazzocchio et al., "Antibacterial Activity of Hydrastis canadensis Extract and Its Major Isolated Alkaloids," *Planta Medica* 67, no. 6 (August 2001): 561–64. doi: 10.1055/s-2001-16493.

20. See his TED Talk at: https://www.ted.com/talks/paul_stamets_on_6_ways_mushrooms_can_save_the_world?language=en.

21. A. G. Guggenheim et al., "Immune Modulation from Five Major Mushrooms: Application to Integrative Oncology," *Integrative Medicine* (Encinitas, CA) 13 no. 1 (February 2014): 32–44. PMID: 26770080.

22. See "Mushrooms and Mycelium Help the Microbiome," http://www.greenmedinfo.com/blog/mushrooms-and-mycelium-help-microbiome.

23. Pallav, Kumar et al., "Effects of Polysaccharopeptide from Trametes versicolor and Amoxicillin on the Gut Microbiome of Healthy Volunteers," *Gut Microbes* 5, no. 4 (July 1, 2014): 458–67. doi: 10.4161/gmic.29558.

24. Dai X et al., "Consuming Lentinula edodes (Shiitake) Mushrooms Daily Improves Human Immunity: A Randomized Dietary Intervention in Healthy Young Adults," *Journal of the American College of Nutrition* 34, no. 6 (April 2015): 478–87. doi: 10.1080/07315724.2014.950391.

25. S. Prabhu and E. K. Poulose, "Silver Nanoparticles: Mechanism of Antimicrobial Action, Synthesis, Medical Applications, and Toxicity Effects," *International Nano Letters* 2 (December 2012): 32. https://doi.org/10.1186/2228-5326-2-32.

26. S. Silver, L. T. Phung, and G. Silver, "Silver as Biocides in Burn and Wound Dressings and Bacterial Resistance to Silver Compounds," *Journal of Industrial Microbiology and Biotechnology* 33, no. 7 (July 2006): 627–34. https://doi.org /10.1007/s10295-006-0139-7.

27. J. S. Kim et al., "Antimicrobial Effects of Silver Nanoparticles," *Nanomedicine* 3, no. 1 (March 2007): 95–101. DOI: 10.1016/j.nano.2006.12.001.

28. M. Bhattacharyya and H. Bradley, "A Case Report of the Use of Nanocrystalline Silver Dressing in the Management of Acute Surgical Site Wound Infected with MRSA to Prevent Cutaneous Necrosis Following Revision Surgery," *International Journal of Lower Extremity Wounds* 7, no. 1 (March 2008): 45–48. doi: 10.1177/1534734607302232.

29. M. Rai et al., "Silver Nanoparticles as a New Generation of Antimicrobials," *Biotechnology Advances* 27, no. 1 (January–February 2009): 76–83. doi: 10.1016 /j.biotechadv.2008.09.002.

30. A. A. Alangari et al., "Honey Is Potentially Effective in the Treatment of Atopic Dermatitis: Clinical and Mechanistic Studies," *Immunity, Inflammation and Disease* 5, no. 2 (June 2017): 190–99. doi: 10.1002/iid3.153.

31. M. Piotrowski et al., "Antimicrobial Effects of Manuka Honey on in Vitro Biofilm Formation by Clostridium difficile," *European Journal of Clinical Microbiology and Infectious Diseases* 36, no. 9 (September 2017): 1661–64. doi: 10.1007/s10096-017 -2980-1.

32. S. L. Giles and R. J. F. Laheij, "Successful Treatment of Persistent Clostridium difficile Infection with Manuka Honey," *International Journal of Antimicrobial Agents* 49, no. 4 (April 2017): 522–23. doi: 10.1016/j.ijantimicag.2017.02.005.

33. S. E. Maddocks et al, "Manuka Honey Inhibits the Development of Streptococcus pyogenes Biofilms and Causes Reduced Expression of Two Fibronectin Binding Proteins," *Microbiology* 158, pt. 3 (March 2012): 781–90. doi: 10.1099/mic .0.053959-0.

34. A. Moussa et al., "Antibacterial Activity of Various Honey Types of Algeria Against Staphylococcus aureus and Streptococcus pyogenes," *Asian Pacific Journal of Tropical Medicine* 5, no. 10 (October 2012): 773–76. doi: 10.1016/S1995 -7645(12)60141-2.

35. "Manuka Honey Helps Combat Urinary Tract Infections," *Nursing Standard* 31, no. 9 (October 2016): 17. doi: 10.7748/ns.31.9.17.s20.

36. M. B. Hussain et al., "In-Vitro Susceptibility of Methicillin-Resistant Stayphylococcus aureus to Honey," *Complementary Therapies in Clinical Practice* 27 (May 2017): 57–60. doi: 10.1016/j.ctcp.2017.04.003.

37. P. M. Kustiawan et al., "Molecular Mechanism of Cardol, Isolated from Trigona incisa Stingless Bee Propolis, Induced Apoptosis in the SW620 Human Colorectal Cancer Cell Line," *BMC Pharmacology and Toxicology* 18, no. 1 (May 4, 2017): 32. doi: 10.1186/s40360-017-0139-4.

38. K. Doi et al., "Chemopreventive Action by Ethanol-Extracted Brazilian Green Propolis on Post-Initiation Phase of Inflammation-associated Rat Colon Tumorigenesis," *In Vivo* 31, no. 2 (March–April 2017): 187–97. doi: 10.21873 /invivo.11044.

39. R. P. Dantas Silva et al., "Antioxidant, Antimicrobial, Antiparasitic, and Cytotoxic Properties of Various Brazilian Propolis Extracts," *PLoS One* 12, no. 3 (March 30, 2017): e0172585. doi: 10.1371/journal.pone.0172585.

40. A. V. Oliveira, "Antibacterial Activity of Propolis Extracts from the South of Portugal," *Pakistan Journal of Pharmaceutical Sciences* 30, no. 1 (January 2017): 1–9. PMID: 28603105.

41. V. Mokhtari et al., "A Review on Various Uses of N-Acetyl Cysteine," *Cell Journal* 19, no. 1 (December 1, 2016): 11–17. PMID: 28367412.

42. Giancarlo Aldini et al., "N-Acetylcysteine as an Antioxidant and Disulphide Breaking Agent: The Reasons Why," *Free Radical Research* 52, Issue 7 (May 2018): 751–62. https://doi.org/10.1080/10715762.2018.1468564.

43. See his book *Inflammation Mastery 4th Edition: The Colorful and Definitive Guide Toward Health and Vitality and away from the Boredom, Risks, Costs, and Inefficacy . . . Immunosuppression, and Polypharmacy* (International College of Human Nutrition and Functional Medicine, 2016).

44. E. S. Wintergerst et al., "Immune-Enhancing Role of Vitamin C and Zinc and Effect on Clinical Conditions," *Annals of Nutrition and Metabolism* 50, no. 2 (2006): 85–94. doi: 10.1159/000090495.

45. S. A. Maggini et al., "A Combination of High-Dose Vitamin C plus Zinc for the Common Cold," *Journal of International Medical Research* 40, no. 1 (2012): 28–42. DOI: 10.1177/147323001204000104.

46. Wintergerst et al., "Immune-Enhancing Role of Vitamin C and Zinc and Effect on Clinical Conditions."

47. See her website: http://drsuzanne.net for how to order her books.

48. B. Kranjčec et al., "D-Mannose Powder for Prophylaxis of Recurrent Urinary Tract Infections in Women: A Randomized Clinical Trial," World Journal of Urology 32, no. 1 (February 2014): 79–84. doi: 10.1007/s00345-013-1091-6.

49. G. J. Ochoa-Brust et al., "Daily Intake of 100 mg Ascorbic Acid as Urinary Tract Infection Prophylactic Agent during Pregnancy," *Acta Obstetrecia et Gynecologica Scandinavica* 86, no. 7 (2007): 783–87. doi: 10.1080/00016340701273189.

50. A. J. Roe et al., "Inhibition of *Escherichia coli* Growth by Acetic Acid: A Problem with Methionine Biosynthesis and Homocysteine Toxicity," *Microbiology* (Reading, U.K.) 148, pt. 7 (July 2002): 2215–22. doi: 10.1099/00221287-148-7 -2215.

51. M. Sienkiewicz et al., "[The Antibacterial Activity of Oregano Essential Oil (Origanum heracleoticum L.) Against Clinical Strains of Escherichia coli and Pseudomonas aeruginosa]," *Med Dosw Mikrobiol* 64, no. 4 (2012) 64(4): 297–307. PMID: 23484421. Article in Polish.

52. C. de Paula Coelho, "Homeopathic Medicine Cantharis Modulates Uropathogenic E. coli (UPEC)-Induced Cystitis in Susceptible Mice," *Cytokine* 92 (April 2017): 103–9. doi: 10.1016/j.cyto.2017.01.014.

53. See Fists of Anger: Meditation for Releasing Anger at http://blog.myvirtualyoga .com/wpcontent/uploads/2017/01/FistsofAnger.pdf.

54. Healthy, Happy, Holy Organization, "Kundalini Yoga for Headaches," https:// www.3ho.org/3ho-lifestyle/health-and-healing/kundalini-yoga-headaches.

55. Healthy, Happy, Holy Organization, "Pranayam to Boost Your Immune System," https://www.3ho.org/articles/pranayam-boost-your-immune-system.

56. Healthy, Happy, Holy Organization, "Ra Ma Da Sa Sa Say So Hung: The Ultimate Healing Tool," https://www.3ho.org/kundalini-yoga/mantra/ra-ma-da-sa-sa-say -so-hung-ultimate-healing-tool.

# BIBLIOGRAPHY

Aldo, Joseph. *Holistic Healing and the Shifting Paradigm: A Transformational Model for Conscious Living Utilizing the Wisdom and Science of Nature.* Privately published.

Barasch, Marc Ian. *The Healing Path: A Soul Approach to Illness.* New York: Tarcher, 1994.

Borysenko, Joan, with Larry Rothstein. *Minding the Body, Mending the Mind.* New York: Bantam, 1988.

Bragdon, Emma, Ph.D. *Shamans and Spiritists: On the Spiritual View of Mental Illness.* Forthcoming.

Breggin, Peter. *Guilt, Shame, and Anxiety: Understanding and Overcoming Negative Emotions.* Amherst, NY: Prometheus, 2014.

———. *Medication Madness: The Rule of Psychiatric Drugs in Cases of Violence, Suicide, and Crime.* New York: St. Martin's, 2008.

———. *Psychiatric Drug Withdrawal: A Guide for Prescribers, Therapists, Patients and Their Families.* New York: Springer, 2013.

———. *Talking Back to Prozac: What Doctors Aren't Telling You About Today's Most Controversial Drug.* New York: St. Martin's, 1994.

———. *Toxic Psychiatry: Why Therapy, Empathy, and Love Must Replace the Drugs, Electroshock, and Biochemical Theories of the "New Psychiatry."* New York: St. Martin's, 1991.

Brogan, Kelly, M.D., and Sofia Brogan Fink. *A Time for Rain.* Privately published, 2018.

Delano, Laura. *Recovering from Psychiatry.* Video.

Dispenza, Joe. *Becoming Supernatural: How Common People Are Doing the Uncommon.* New York: Hay House, 2017.

———. *You Are the Placebo: Making Your Mind Matter.* New York: Hay House, 2015.

Eisenstein, Charles. *The More Beautiful World Our Hearts Know Is Possible.* Berkeley, CA: North Atlantic, 2013.

———. *The Yoga of Eating: Transcending Diets and Dogma to Nourish the Natural Self.* Washington, DC: New Trends, 2003.

Estés, Clarissa Pinkola. *Women Who Run with the Wolves: Myths and Stories of the Wild Woman Archetype.* New York: Ballantine, 1992.

Frankl, Viktor. *Man's Search for Meaning.* Boston: Beacon, 1959.

Hall, Will. *Harm Reduction Guide to Coming Off Psychiatric Drugs.* New York: Icarus Project and Northampton, MA: Freedom Center, 2007. Available online for free: https://willhall.net/files/ComingOffPsychDrugsHarmReductGuide2Edonline.pdf.

Jagat, Guru. *Invincible Living: The Power of Yoga, the Energy of Breath, and Other Tools for a Radiant Life.* New York: HarperCollins, 2017.

Kaur, Mahankirn. *Three Min Start: 22 Simple Techniques to Radically Improve Mood and Performance*. Los Angeles: Boundlotus, 2012.

Khalsa, Dharma Singh and Cameron Stauth. *Meditation as Medicine: Activate the Power of Your Natural Healing Force*. New York: Simon and Schuster, 2001.

Khalsa, Dharma Singh and Darryl O'Keefe. *The Kundalini Yoga Experience: Bringing Body, Mind, and Spirit Together*. New York: Simon and Schuster, 2002.

Levy, Paul. *The Quantum Revelation: A Radical Synthesis of Science and Spirituality*. New York: SelectBooks, 2018.

Lipton, Bruce. *The Biology of Belief: Unleashing the Power of Consciousness, Matter & Miracles*. New York: Hay House, 2005.

Masters, Robert Augustus. *Spiritual Bypassing: When Spirituality Disconnects Us from What Really Matters*. Berkeley, CA: North Atlantic, 2010.

Moncrieff, Joanna. *The Bitterest Pills: The Troubling Story of Antipsychotic Drugs*. New York: Palgrave Macmillan, 2013.

Northrup, Christiane. *Dodging Energy Vampires: An Empath's Guide to Evading Relationships That Drain You and Restoring Your Health and Power*. New York: Hay House, 2018.

Perel, Esther. *Mating in Captivity: Unlocking Erotic Intelligence*. New York: HarperCollins, 2017.

Pert, Candace. *Molecules of Emotion: The Science Behind Mind-Body Medicine*. New York: Simon and Schuster, 1997.

Shannahoff-Khalsa, David. *Sacred Therapies: The Kundalini Yoga Meditation Handbook for Mental Health*. New York: W. W. Norton, 2012.

Sheldrake, Rupert. *Morphic Resonance: The Nature of Formative Causation*. New York: Tarcher, 1981.

———. *A New Science of Life: The Hypothesis of Morphic Resonance*. Rochester, VT: Inner Traditions, 1995.

———. *The Presence of the Past: Morphic Resonance and the Memory of Nature*. Rochester, VT: Inner Traditions, 1988.

———. *The Science Delusion: Freeing the Spirit of Enquiry*. London: Hodder and Stoughton, 2012.

Singer, Michael. *The Surrender Experiment: My Journey into Life's Perfection*. New York: Harmony, 2015.

———. *The Untethered Soul: The Journey Beyond Yourself*. Oakland, CA: New Harbinger, 2007.

Thomashauer, Regena (Mama Gena). *Mama Gena's Marriage Manual: Stop Being a Good Wife, Start Being a Sister Goddess!* New York: Simon and Schuster, 2005.

———. *Mama Gena's Owner's and Operator's Guide to Men*. New York: Simon and Schuster 2002.

———. *Mama Gena's School of Womanly Arts: Using the Power of Pleasure to Have Your Way with the World*. New York: Simon and Schuster 2002.

———. *Pussy: A Reclamation*. New York: Hay House, 2016.

Tsabary, Shefali. *The Awakened Family: How to Raise Empowered, Resilient, and Conscious Children*. New York: Penguin, 2016.

Van der Kolk, Bessel. *The Body Keeps the Score: Brain, Mind, and Body in the Healing of Trauma*. New York: Penguin, 2014.

Vasquez, Alex. *Inflammation Mastery 4th Edition: The Colorful and Definitive Guide Toward Health and Vitality and away from the Boredom, Risks, Costs, and Inefficacy . . . Immunosuppression, and Polypharmacy.* International College of Human Nutrition and Functional Medicine, 2016.

Watts, Alan. *Does it Matter? Essays on Man's Relation to Materiality.* Novato, CA: New World Library, 2007.

————. "Psychedelics and Religious Experience," *California Law Review* 56, issue 1, article 6 (January 1968). Berkeley, CA: Berkeley Law Scholarship Repository.

Weller, Francis. *The Wild Edge of Sorrow: Rituals of Renewal and the Sacred Work of Grief.* Berkeley, CA: North Atlantic, 2015.

Whitaker, Robert. *Anatomy of an Epidemic: Magic Bullets, Psychiatric Drugs, and the Astonishing Rise of Mental Illness in America.* New York: Crown, 2010.

————. *Mad in America: Bad Science, Bad Medicine, and the Enduring Mistreatment of the Mentally Ill.* New York: Perseus, 2001.

Whitaker, Robert (with Lisa Cosgrove). *Psychiatry Under the Influence: Institutional Corruption, Social Injury, and Prescriptions for Reform.* New York: Palgrave Macmillan, 2015.

Yogi Bhajan. *I Am a Woman: Creative, Sacred and Invincible—Essential Kriyas for Women in the Aquarian Age.* Santa Cruz, CA: Kundalini Research Institute, 2009.

————. *Kriya: Yoga Sets, Meditations and Classic Kriyas.* Santa Cruz, CA: Kundalini Research Institute, 2013.

————. *Rebirthing: Breath, Vitality, Strength.* Santa Cruz, CA: Kundalini Research Institute, 2011.

Yogi Bhajan and Hari Jot Kaur. *Praana, Praanee, Praanayam.* Santa Cruz, CA: Kundalini Research Institute, 2006.

# INDEX

# B

# C

# ACKNOWLEDGMENTS

In gratitude to my new family at Hay House, including the savvy and sage Patty Gift, the intrepid and humble Reid Tracy, and the gentle and brilliant Anne Barthel.

In gratitude to Nancy Marriott for her unstoppable crystalline mind, and for walking her path right onto my own so that we could create this manuscript together in perfect complementarity.

In gratitude to Bonnie Solow, Kristin Loberg, and Karen Rinaldi for standing with me in the creation of *A Mind of Your Own* and then loving me enough to let me go.

In gratitude to Sayer, for showing up in this lifetime as the most breathtaking embodiment of the sacred masculine I could ever have dreamt. Thank you for breaking my false self into a thousand pieces and mending the cracks with gold as I create the self I long to be, in devotional honoring of the godhead you are.

In gratitude to my maternal lineage, my mother, Marusca, my Nonnie, Bianca, and beyond, for doing the absolute best work you could to sustain the fire of creation that burns within the woman.

In gratitude to my family of origin, Marusca, Ron, Brendan, and Sara, and to Mattie, and the Hatfield, Tognetti, Ojjeh, and Fink families for loving me in exactly the ways that I have needed in order for me to awaken to a fuller embrace of my self.

In gratitude to Sofia, goddess of wisdom, and an endless source of wit, creativity, and depth.

In gratitude to Lucia, goddess of light, empath and liberator of wild emotions for the betterment of all.

In gratitude to Andy Fink for making it impossible to feel anything but love for you, always.

In gratitude to Lisa, Mia, Bella, Sienna, and Dottie Ji for welcoming me into your hearts.

In gratitude to Tahra Collins for honoring our soul contract to hold each other with ferocity and unconditional love through transformation and for showing up, every day, as the radiant angel you are. There is no me without you.

In gratitude to Louise Kuo for wading around in the muck with me, and for turning our activism sacred.

In gratitude to Swaranpal for being the mother I needed when I did, and the sister I'll need now and forever.

In gratitude to Leela Lorenzoni for your steadfastness, honesty, and humble support, your devotion to this mission, and your pure heart.

In gratitude to Alyssa Siefert for blessing me with your endless gifts, but specifically with your heart wisdom, your curious mind, your yes to every turn on our shared path toward spiritualizing science, and your critical eyes on this manuscript.

In gratitude to Katie Hess for your magic, your flowers, and your golden heart.

In gratitude to Sarah Kamrath for your truth-telling, your smile, and your love of the light.

In gratitude to Christiane Northrup for the gift of your wisdom, your radiance, and your warm hand on the dark path.

In gratitude to Carrie-Anne Moss for your support and your deep femininity, always nearby.

In gratitude to Whitney Burrell for loving me through my many iterations, for your brilliant mind and your open heart.

In gratitude to James Maskell and Gabe Hoffman for holding a vision for the future of medicine and including me in it.

In gratitude to Mary Beth Gonzalez and Dr. Linda Isaacs for supporting Nick's legacy and for helping me to find my place in it.

In gratitude to Charles Eisenstein for your soul-companionship and the humble channeling of truths that bring me closer to home.

In gratitude to Maya Shetreat-Klein for holding the space of witches becoming, with me.

In gratitude to Astrid Schmidt for honoring this new story of mental health with me, and for your wisdom and depth of heart.

In gratitude to Suzanne Moscovitch for honoring our karmic destiny in support of one another's healing, and in service to the world.

In gratitude to Scott McDermott for granting me the gift of your presence in my life, with your kaleidoscopic talents, deep kindness, refined sensitivity, and dedication to sharing this message far and wide.

In gratitude to Tracy Bertrand for your laughs, your commitment, and your support.

In gratitude to Jamie Davidson for your courage to heal in order to spread light, with us, in a way that only you can.

In gratitude to Mingtong Gu for sharing your radiant joy with me and bringing the promise of quantum healing to this country.

In gratitude to Joseph Aldo for always giving me the deep feeling of being seen and understood.

In gratitude to Alison Birnbaum for introducing me to my inner child and many of the related concepts in this book, and for holding the container for the transformation of generations of family karma.

In gratitude to Rachel Koenig, Shiva Schiff, and Angelica Lemke for supporting my healing journey and the transformation of my fire into the smoldering cauldron of femininity.

In gratitude to Natalie Christensen for reminding me how to apply my work with women to my work as a mother.

In gratitude to Ron and Katya for holding exquisite space for my contact with the divine.

In gratitude to Louisa and Ilan Bohm for your dedication to the heart-opening path of self-discovery.

In gratitude to Luis Molinar and Claudia Morales for your warmth, your cacao, and our shared love of transcendence.

In gratitude to Belinda Inman and to Marguerite Insolia for gracefully channeling the spiritual support I sometimes needed to be reminded was there.

To the newest additions to my coven, Kukuwa, Daniela, Nikki, Stacey, Rebecca, Tatiana, Mitzi, Pema, Vero, Susan, and the Waldorf community. Our connections are evidence that I am indeed on the path.

To all of our VMR participants, ambassadors, coaches, community managers past and present, and to all of my patients, and to all of you who have stood with me in service of a new story. I simply couldn't have seen a path forward without your light.

# ABOUT THE AUTHOR

Kelly Brogan, M.D., is a holistic women's health psychiatrist, author of the *New York Times* best-selling book *A Mind of Your Own* and the children's book *A Time for Rain*, and coeditor of the landmark textbook *Integrative Therapies for Depression*. She completed her psychiatric training and fellowship at NYU Medical Center after graduating from Cornell University Medical College, and has a B.S. from MIT in systems neuroscience. She is board certified in psychiatry, psychosomatic medicine, and integrative holistic medicine and is specialized in a root-cause resolution approach to psychiatric syndromes and symptoms. She is a certified KRI Kundalini Yoga teacher and a mother of two.

Website: kellybroganmd.com

# Hay House Titles of Related Interest

*YOU CAN HEAL YOUR LIFE, the movie,* starring Louise Hay & Friends
(available as a 1-DVD program, an expanded 2-DVD set,
and an online streaming video)
Learn more at www.hayhouse.com/louise-movie

*THE SHIFT, the movie,* starring Dr. Wayne W. Dyer
(available as a 1-DVD program, an expanded 2-DVD set,
and an online streaming video)
Learn more at www.hayhouse.com/the-shift-movie

———

*DODGING ENERGY VAMPIRES: An Empath's Guide to
Evading Relationships That Drain You and Restoring
Your Health and Power,* by Christiane Northrup, M.D.

*THE MINDBODY SELF: How Longevity Is Culturally Learned and the
Causes of Health Are Inherited,* by Dr. Mario Martinez

*PUSSY: A Reclamation,* by Regena Thomashauer

*YOU ARE THE PLACEBO: Making Your Mind Matter,*
by Dr. Joe Dispenza

———

All of the above are available at your local bookstore,
or may be ordered by contacting Hay House (seenextpage).

We hope you enjoyed this Hay House book. If you'd like to receive our online catalog featuring additional information on Hay House books and products, or if you'd like to find out more about the Hay Foundation, please contact:

Hay House, Inc., P.O. Box 5100, Carlsbad, CA 92018-5100
(760) 431-7695 or (800) 654-5126
(760) 431-6948 (fax) or (800) 650-5115 (fax)
www.hayhouse.com® • www.hayfoundation.org

———

*Published in Australia by:* Hay House Australia Pty. Ltd.,
18/36 Ralph St., Alexandria NSW 2015
*Phone:* 612-9669-4299 • *Fax:* 612-9669-4144
www.hayhouse.com.au

*Published in the United Kingdom by:* Hay House UK, Ltd.,
The Sixth Floor, Watson House, 54 Baker Street, London W1U 7BU
*Phone:* +44 (0)20 3927 7290 • *Fax:* +44 (0)20 3927 7291
www.hayhouse.co.uk

*Published in India by:* Hay House Publishers India,
Muskaan Complex, Plot No. 3, B-2, Vasant Kunj, New Delhi 110 070
*Phone:* 91-11-4176-1620 • *Fax:* 91-11-4176-1630
www.hayhouse.co.in

———

## Access New Knowledge.
## Anytime. Anywhere.

Learn and evolve at your own pace
with the world's leading experts.

www.hayhouseU.com

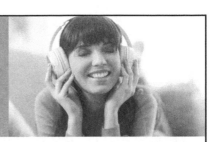
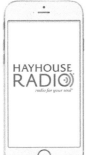